DEBATES IN MEDICINE
Volume 1

DEBATES IN MEDICINE

Editorial Board

Editor-in-Chief
Gary Gitnick, M.D.
Professor, Department of Medicine
UCLA School of Medicine
Center for Health Sciences
Los Angeles, California

Associate Editors
H. Verdain Barnes, M.D.
Professor and Chairman
Department of Medicine
Wright State University
School of Medicine
Dayton, Ohio

Thomas P. Duffy, M.D.
Professor of Medicine
Section of Hematology
Department of Internal Medicine
Yale University School of Medicine
New Haven, Connecticut

Nicholas J. Fortuin, M.D.
Professor of Medicine
The Johns Hopkins University
School of Medicine
Baltimore, Maryland

Volume 1 • 1988

Year Book Medical Publishers, Inc.
Chicago • London • Boca Raton

International Standard Serial Number: 0887-218X
International Standard Book Number: 0-8151-3600-5

Sponsoring Editor: James F. Shanahan
Assistant Director, Manuscript Services: Frances M. Perveiler
Production Project Manager: Max Perez
Proofroom Supervisor: Shirley E. Taylor

Contributors

Allen C. Alfrey, M.D.
Professor of Medicine
Department of Medicine
University of Colorado
Health Sciences Center
Chief, Renal Medicine
Veterans Administration Medical Center
Denver, Colorado

David A. August, M.D.
Assistant Professor
Department of Surgery
Division of Surgical Oncology
Yale University School of Medicine
New Haven, Connecticut

Henry R. Black, M.D.
Associate Professor of Medicine
Department of Medicine
Yale University School of Medicine
New Haven, Connecticut

Gary L. Davis, M.D.
Associate Professor of Medicine
Division of Gastroenterology, Hepatology and Nutrition
University of Florida
College of Medicine
Gainesville, Florida

Thomas P. Duffy, M.D.
Professor of Medicine
Section of Hematology
Department of Internal Medicine
Yale University School of Medicine
New Haven, Connecticut

Paul H. Duray, M.D.
Director, Division of Anatomic Pathology
Fox Chase Cancer Center
Philadelphia, Pennsylvania

Marc S. Ernstoff, M.D.

Assistant Professor of Medicine
Division of Medical Oncology
Department of Medicine
University of Pittsburgh School of Medicine
Pittsburgh Cancer Institute
Pittsburgh, Pennsylvania

Rosemarie Fisher, M.D.

Associate Professor of Medicine
Gastroenterology Unit
Yale University School of Medicine
New Haven, Connecticut

Kim Goldenberg, M.D.

Associate Professor and Director
General Internal Medicine Division
Department of Medicine
Wright State University School of Medicine
Dayton, Ohio

Barry H. Greenberg, M.D.

Professor of Medicine
Director, Coronary Care Unit
Oregon Health Sciences University
Portland, Oregon

Richard J. Gusberg, M.D.

Associate Professor of Surgery
Department of General and Vascular Surgery
Yale University School of Medicine
New Haven, Connecticut

Karl E. Hammermeister, M.D.

Professor of Medicine
University of Colorado
Health Sciences Center
Chief of Cardiology
Veterans Administration Medical Center
Denver, Colorado

Robert P. Heaney, M.D.

John A. Creighton University Professor
Creighton University
Omaha, Nebraska

D. M. Hegsted, M.D.
Professor of Nutrition Emeritus
Harvard Schools of Public Health and Medicine
New England Regional Primate Research Center
Southborough, Massachusetts

Angela R. Holder, LL.M.
Counsel for Medicolegal Affairs
Yale University School of Medicine and Yale-New Haven Hospital
Clinical Professor of Pediatrics (Law)
Yale University School of Medicine
New Haven, Connecticut

Thomas Hostetter, M.D.
Associate Professor of Medicine
Director, Section of Renal Disease
Department of Medicine
University of Minnesota Hospitals
Minneapolis, Minnesota

Norman M. Kaplan, M.D.
Professor of Internal Medicine
Chief, Hypertension Division
Department of Internal Medicine
University of Texas Southwestern Medical School
Dallas, Texas

John M. Kirkwood, M.D.
Chief, Section of Medical Oncology
Department of Medicine
University of Pittsburgh Cancer Institute
Pittsburgh, Pennsylvania

Marvin Moser, M.D.
Clinical Professor of Medicine
Department of Internal Medicine
Yale University School of Medicine
New Haven, Connecticut

Thomas J. Ryan, M.D.
Professor of Medicine
Department of Medicine
Boston University Medical School
Chief of Cardiology
The University Hospital
Boston, Massachusetts

Evangelista Sagnelli, M.D.
Associate Professor of Clinical Virology
Clinic of Infectious Diseases
First School of Medicine
University of Naples
Naples, Italy

Arthur Selzer, M.D.
Clinical Professor of Medicine
University of California at San Francisco
Clinical Professor Emeritus
Stanford University School of Medicine
Stanford, California

John F. Setaro, M.D.
Westchester Hypertension Foundation Fellow
Department of Medicine
Yale University School of Medicine
New Haven, Connecticut

Linda Titus-Ernstoff
Department of Epidemiology
Graduate School of Public Health
University of Pittsburgh
Pittsburgh, Pennsylvania

Anthony C. Wooley, M.D.
Instructor, Renal Division
Department of Medicine
University of Minnesota Hospitals
Minneapolis, Minnesota

Preface

The study of medicine evolved out of controversy. It should not surprise us, then, to find that scientific literature is based on a history of controversy, nor that controversy remains such a fundamental part of this discipline. Regardless of our area of clinical or laboratory study and regardless of whether we are discussing treatment, causation, or pathophysiology, there will be differences of opinion, conflicting data, and contradictory concepts. Through the thoughtful study of all sides of these controversial issues, the astute clinician or student can become exceptionally well versed in medicine.

This volume devotes a chapter to each of ten prominent controversies. The associate editors and I have chosen contributing authors who are experts in particular areas, and have instructed each to provide the very best case to be made for a given position. In some instances, as is sometimes the case with oral debates, authors have been asked to present a view that may be opposite to the one they espouse. However, in most cases, the positions presented herein are consistent with the views expressed by the authors in their previous publications and public statements.

At the end of each chapter, we provide editorial remarks in the way of a brief summary and an evaluation of the strengths and weaknesses of the arguments. Our comments should also be taken as opinion, which has been said to be composed of a minimum of fact combined with prejudice and imagination. Nevertheless, we have tried to tie together the differing opinions and guide the reader through our current state of ignorance.

I am indebted to the associate editors and contributing authors who diligently developed their arguments and who were exceptionally cooperative in efficiently and promptly sending their chapters to me.

I wish to thank the associate editors who worked closely with me in the development of this volume. They are H. Verdain Barnes, M.D., Thomas P. Duffy, M.D., and Nicholas Fortuin, M.D. I wish to thank Mrs. Susan Dashe, who coordinated the development of this volume, and Mr. James Shanahan of Year Book Medical Publishers, Inc.; his support was of great assistance. Most readers will find opinions in this volume with which they greatly disagree. It is our hope that this disagreement will stimulate thought and insight, that knowledge of all sides of the controversies will expand basic knowledge of the diseases discussed, and that the reader will not only learn from but will also enjoy this book.

Gary Gitnick, M.D.

Contents

Coronary Bypass Surgery or Angioplasty Should Be Used for Patients With Stable Symptoms

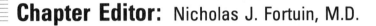

Chapter Editor: Nicholas J. Fortuin, M.D.

Affirmative: Karl E. Hammermeister, M.D.
Professor of Medicine, University of
Colorado, Health Sciences Center; Chief of
Cardiology, Veterans Administration Medical
Center, Denver, Colorado

Negative: Thomas J. Ryan, M.D.
Professor of Medicine, Department of
Medicine, Boston University Medical School;
Chief of Cardiology, The University
Hospital, Boston, Massachusetts

Debates in Medicine 1:2–63, 1988
©1988, Year Book Medical Publishers, Inc.
0887-218X/88/01-002-029-$04.00

Affirmative
Karl E. Hammermeister, M.D.

The answer to this problem is clearly yes—in some patients. The problem has been to determine through valid studies which subgroups of patients will benefit through prolongation of life and/or improvement of symptoms and functional capacity. A second, related problem has been to develop and validate inexpensive, safe, noninvasive techniques to identify such patients. The solutions to both of these problems are only partially known. This essay will discuss the available information relevant to the first problem.

First, it might be well to define what is meant by stable symptoms. Some patients will be severely limited by ischemic myocardial symptoms and yet be in a stable phase of their disease. Because there is abundant evidence that revascularization either by angioplasty in selected patients or by coronary bypass graft surgery (CABG) can improve symptoms and increase exercise capacity, there is little controversy about what to do in such patients; a revascularization procedure should be recommended if the anatomy is suitable and the operative risk acceptable. The greatest difficulty lies with those patients whose ischemic myocardial symptoms are mild or even nonexistent. Proponents of an aggressive approach point to the relatively high incidence of stable, mild symptoms or no symptoms in patients experiencing sudden cardiac death.

There are three major reasons to recommend any therapy: (1) to improve symptoms, (2) to preserve health and functional capacity, and (3) to prolong life. The remainder of this essay will concentrate primarily on the third indication, as patients with mild or no symptoms are unlikely to experience improvement, and little is known about the second indication. Because there are few or no data on the effect of angioplasty on survival, the discussion will concentrate on the results of CABG.

Our modern understanding of coronary death being due to ischemia arose following the description by Herrick in 1912[1] of acute myocardial infarction as being the result of obstruction of the coronary artery and the observation by Wood and Wolferth in 1931[2] that angina pectoris is associated with electrocardiographic evidence of ischemia. Soon thereafter, the first surgical procedures to correct myocardial ischemia were attempted. Although procedures such as pericardial poudrage with talc to stimulate anastomoses between the pericardium and epicardium, wrapping the omentum around the heart to provide blood flow to the epicardial surface from the mesenteric vessels, and internal mammary artery ligation were reported to result in symptomatic relief in the majority of patients, there were few controlled studies. The exception to this statement is the internal mammary artery ligation, where two controlled, blinded studies using sham operations showed the procedure to have no benefit.[3, 4] These are two of the few instances in which it has been possible to use blinding and sham procedures to control for the placebo effect of a surgical procedure, something none of the modern randomized trials of CABG have been able to do. These procedures, like the internal mammary artery implantation procedure (Vineberg procedure), were doomed to failure because the amount of increase (if any) in blood supply to the myocardium was small in relation to the need.

However, soon after the introduction of the saphenous vein aortocoronary bypass operation by Favalaro in 1967,[5] it was possible to demonstrate that the surgically created conduits could carry 50% or more of the myocardial blood supply. This, coupled with the fact that the operation could be performed at a low operative mortality, led to the widespread conviction in the early 1970s that this was a life-saving procedure. This conviction was reinforced by nonrandomized, observational studies showing that virtually all subgroups except those with single-vessel disease involving the right or circumflex coronary arteries had improved survival with surgical therapy as compared with medical therapy.[6] It was not widely recognized then that this and many other similar studies did not adequately take into account differences between medically and surgically treated patients.

Needless to say, there was much disappointment and controversy when the results of the first large randomized trial comparing survival of medical and surgical therapy in patients with stable angina, the VA Cooperative Study, showed improved survival only in the small subgroup with left main coronary artery stenosis.[7, 8]

This introduction has deliberately set the scene by picking studies showing extremes in their results: (1) the very early Cleveland Clinic study purporting improved survival in the majority of patients operated on, and (2) the first reports of the VA Cooperative Study showing survival benefit only in a minority of their patients. It is now widely recognized that selection bias (selecting better-risk patients for surgery) strongly influences the outcome of nonrandomized studies, particularly if little or no attempt has been made to adjust for baseline differences. However, it is not generally accepted that randomized trials may present too conservative a viewpoint, primarily because the patients selected are not representative of the general population of patients with coronary heart disease being considered for CABG. This latter theme will be developed in more detail after presentation of outcome data from the four large randomized trials comparing surgical vs. medical therapy for coronary artery disease (CAD); these randomized trial data will be supplemented with data from observational studies where adjustments for baseline differences have been made.

Stable Angina Pectoris

Left Main Coronary Artery Obstruction

The first large, randomized, controlled study testing the hypothesis that surgical relief of myocardial ischemia prolongs life was the VA Cooperative Study. The first report of outcome from this study was on the relatively small subgroup with left main coronary artery stenosis (diameter reduction > 50%), showing dramatically improved survival in the surgically treated group.[7] All subsequent studies in which this issue was seriously addressed have confirmed the result of the VA Cooperative Study. It is now generally accepted that patients with significant left main coronary artery stenosis should have CABG, regardless of whether symptoms are present, providing that the patient's general medical condition allows the surgery to be accomplished at a reasonable operative risk.

Single-Vessel CAD

All of the randomized trials and most of the observational studies show no improvement in survival in patients with single-vessel disease, because survival of patients with single-vessel disease is not appreciably different from that of the general population of similar age. The controversy over the effect on survival is in the patients with two- and three-vessel disease. Even here there is abundant evidence that CABG relieves symptoms that cannot otherwise be controlled with medical therapy. Most will agree that limiting angina refractory to medical therapy in patients with graftable distal vessels and who are acceptable operative risks should be treated with CABG or percutaneous transluminal coronary angioplasty (PTCA) if appropriate.

Three-Vessel Coronary Artery Disease

At first glance the randomized trial data concerning patients with three-vessel disease may seem confusing and conflicting. The initial report of the VA Cooperative Study showed no survival benefit for operative therapy of three-vessel disease,[8] whereas a later report did[9]; the European Coronary Surgery Study (ECSS) showed a marked reduction in mortality in the patients with three-vessel disease who were bypassed,[10] but the Coronary Artery Surgery Study (CASS) conducted in the United States and Canada showed no overall difference in survival.[11] Even now the conflict in the results of the European and VA studies on the one hand and CASS on the other is not easily resolved. Let us consider some of the issues.

The initial report of the VA study in 1977 showing no difference in survival between medical and surgical therapy was labeled by its authors as preliminary[8] but was regarded by many at that time as the "final word."

In a subsequent analysis, the VA investigators eliminated the data for the three hospitals with an average 23% operative mortality (which contributed only 13% of the patients to the study) and found a statistically significant improvement in survival for surgically treated three-vessel disease for patients operated on at the ten remaining hospitals, with a 3.3% operative mortality.[9] This post hoc analysis of a subset of patients selected on the basis of outcome clearly violates an important study design principle. On the other hand, an operative mortality of 23% is extraordinarily high, even for that era, and suggests technical problems in the performance of the surgery. Thus, I maintain that there is some validity to this analysis.

Other subgroup analyses from the VA study have shown improved survival with operative therapy in an angiographic high-risk subgroup and the high-risk tercile defined by noninvasive criteria.[10] The angiographic high-risk patients had three-vessel disease and abnormal left ventricular function; this group is similar both in angiographic characteristics and treatment effect to the group with three-vessel disease and abnormal left ventricular function in CASS. The noninvasive risk terciles were defined by four noninvasive variables: history of hypertension, prior myocardial infarction, ST segment depression on the resting electrocardiogram, and New York Heart Association functional class. The patients in the high-risk tercile who had two or three of the strongest risk factors (ST segment depression, history of myocardial infarction, history of hypertension) had significantly better survival when treated surgically. Thus, although the preliminary report of the VA study showed no survival benefit, longer follow-up and subsequent analyses have been able to identify several subgroups where survival is improved by CABG. It is important to note that the survival differences in all subgroups where surgery initially provided better survival appear to be narrowing after 8 years of follow-up.[10] This reemphasizes the fact that this is a palliative operation; the basic pathologic process, obstructive atherosclerosis, continues to advance in the native coronary arteries and develops de novo in the vein grafts.

The ECSS is a randomized trial comparing medical with surgical therapy in 768 men under the age of 65 years with angina pectoris of 3 months' duration or longer.[11] Patients with severe angina not controllable medically, or left ventricular ejection fraction less than 0.50, or single-vessel CAD were excluded. An exact comparison of symptomatic status between patients in the European study and the VA study or CASS is not possible because of the way the data were recorded; nevertheless, it seems likely that the majority of patients in this study may have had mild angina because of the exclusion of those with medically uncontrollable angina. Thus, in this regard the ECSS patients appear to have been similar to the CASS patients. Yet the results of the two studies are markedly different. The European study has shown a 67% reduction in mortality at 5 years for the surgically treated patients with three-vessel disease (6%) compared with medically treated patients (18%). This marked difference remains at 8 years (8% and 23%, respectively). Subgroup analyses showed that the survival benefit was seen in patients with left anterior descending coronary artery obstruction, but not in those without; and in patients with 1.5-mm ST segment depression or more on exercise testing, but not in those with less exertional ST segment depression.[11]

The CASS began entering patients into the randomized trial in 1975 to test the hypothesis that operative therapy would prolong survival in patients with few or no myocardial ischemic symptoms.[12] During the next 3½ years 780 patients with mild angina (Canadian Heart Association classification I or II) or no angina 3 weeks or more after an acute myocardial infarction were entered. A registry was maintained of all patients with suspected CAD undergoing coronary arteriography at the 15 participating centers; almost 25,000 patients were entered into the registry. Thus, the first important point to consider is that the randomized trial patients constituted only 3% of the patients undergoing coronary arteriography for suspected CAD; in other words, this was a highly select group. The 6-year survival of the medically treated patients of 90% is essentially the same as that of the general population of similar age. To further emphasize the low risk of the CASS patients, it is useful to compare the mortality of the medically treated patients with three-vessel disease at 5 years with other studies: 8% in CASS but 18% in the European study and 25% in the VA study. These differences in mortality are all the more significant because the European study required a normal left ventricular ejection fraction (>0.50) and only a 50% reduction in diameter as a significant stenosis, whereas CASS included patients with ejection fractions down to 0.35 and required a 70% reduction in luminal diameter. Thus, it is apparent to me that the CASS investigators have in some way selected an extremely low-risk group of patients for randomization. Unfortunately, the characteristics that differentiate these low-risk patients in CASS from the higher-risk patients in the VA and European studies are not readily apparent. Nonetheless, it is not surprising that there was no overall difference in survival between medically and surgically treated patients in the CASS randomized trial. However, subgroup analyses have shown a statistically significant survival benefit for patients with three-vessel disease and moderately abnormal left ventricular function (ejection fraction, 0.35 to 0.50).[13] Improved survival with surgical therapy has not been seen in any other subgroup defined by the extent of CAD and left ventricular ejection fraction. The differences in results between CASS and the European study are not readily explained by known differences in patient characteristics. I believe that more credence should be given to the European study than it has received to date in this country. It may well be that the results of CASS are less representative of the "real world" as suggested by the extraordinary degree of selectivity of patients in the randomized trial and because of the exceptionally good outcome of these patients, both medically and surgically treated.

Two-Vessel Disease

None of the large randomized trials has shown improved survival with surgical therapy in the overall group of patients with two-vessel CAD. However, when ECSS patients were reclassified according to 75% or greater luminal reduction as the definition of a significant stenosis, the subgroup with two-vessel disease, one of which was the left anterior descending coronary artery, experienced improved survival with surgical therapy.[14] The 8-year mortality of surgically treated patients in this group was 10%, compared with 21% for medically treated patients (P = .013). In the subgroup with two-vessel disease without left anterior descending coronary artery involvement, there was no difference in mortality between the medically treated (14%) and surgically treated (11%) patients at 8 years.

Other Subgroup Analyses

We have explored the possible survival benefit of CABG in subgroups of patients from the nonrandomized Seattle Heart Watch Coronary Arteriography Registry using multivariate statistical techniques to adjust for baseline differences between medically and surgically treated patients.[15–17] Though this type of analysis does not carry the scientific strength of the randomized trial design, it does have certain advantages. First, the population studied is more likely to be representative of the "real world" because there is much less selectivity than occurs with entry of patients into a randomized trial. For example, the 1,880 surgically treated patients in this registry represent about 95% of all patients receiving CABG in Seattle between 1969 and 1974. A second advantage is that the size of the population studied allows multiple subgroup analyses. These analyses suggested that surgery improved survival in patients with two- or three-vessel disease but not single-vessel disease; in patients over the age of 48 but not under; in patients without cardiomegaly but not in those with; in patients without peripheral vascular disease but not in those with; in patients without a history of congestive heart failure but not in those with; in patients without diabetes but not in those with; and in patients without ventricular arrhythmia on the resting electrocardiogram but not in those with.[17]

Similar types of analyses have been done using the registry patients in CASS. These observational analyses of nonrandomized patients have suggested improved survival with surgical therapy in the two highest-risk quartiles of patients over the age of 65[18] and patients with ventricular aneurysm falling into moderate- and high-risk subgroups.[19] When sudden death was used as an end point, the CASS investigators used the observational data analysis technique to show benefit with surgical therapy for the three highest-risk quartiles in the registry.[20]

Conclusions

Coronary artery disease carries with it marked variability in prognosis. The major determinants are the amount of remaining viable myocardium and the extent to which that myocardium is jeopardized by coronary atherosclerosis. Predicted survival of patients with CAD can vary from that of the general age-matched U.S. population for patients with single-vessel disease, to an estimated 1% probability of 6-year survival for a patient with three-vessel disease, ejection fraction of 0.30, cardiomegaly, and left ventricular hypertrophy.[21] A logical deduction from this prognostic information is that there will be some patients whose prognosis is so good that improved survival would not be seen with any form of therapy short of the "fountain of youth." Similarly, one would expect to find a group of patients with such advanced atherosclerosis and its consequences that revascularization would be unlikely to improve survival. However, in between lies a substantial group of patients who will have improved survival with revascularization. There is little question that patients with left main CAD and those with three-vessel disease and moderately abnormal left ventricular function experience improved survival with CABG. Similarly, there is little controversy over the lack of survival benefit in patients with single-vessel disease or in those with two-vessel disease not involving the left anterior descending coronary artery. There remains considerable controversy about patients with three-vessel disease and normal left ventricular function and those with two-vessel disease involving the left anterior descending coronary artery. Here, clinical judgment and common sense need to be used rather than the rigid application of the results of one or another of the randomized trials. One should avoid being tied too tightly to the one-, two-, three-vessel disease concept. A more physiologically sensible concept is that which considers the amount of myocardium at jeopardy and the proportion of that which can be revascularized. Some patients with three-vessel disease may have only a small amount of myocardium at jeopardy if two of the three vessels are totally occluded and the supplied myocardium has already infarcted. Similarly, some patients with two-vessel disease may present with a major portion of the left ventricular myocardium at jeopardy. The likelihood of successful revascularization has to be taken into consideration as well. A posterior descending coronary artery with multiple stenoses throughout its length is much less likely to have successful long-term revascularization than if the vessel had a single tight stenosis at its origin.

The answer to the question "Should coronary bypass surgery be performed in patients with stable symptoms?" is clearly yes—in some patients. Sufficient information is currently available from randomized trials and observational data analyses, which, when combined with good clinical judgment, will allow the selection of patients who are likely to experience improved survival. Still, one must not confuse improvement of survival with improvement of symptoms as indications for coronary artery revascularization. Many patients whose survival will not be prolonged still should have CABG or angioplasty, because their symptoms cannot be adequately controlled with medical therapy.

References

1. Herrick JR: Clinical features of sudden obstruction of the coronary arteries. *JAMA* 1912; 59:2015–2019.
2. Wood FC, Wolferth CC: Angina pectoris: The clinical and electrocardiographic phenomena of the attack and their comparison with the effects of experimental temporary coronary occlusion. *Arch Intern Med* 1931; 47:339–365.
3. Cobb LA, Thomas GI, Dillard DH, et al: An evaluation of internal-mammary-artery ligation by a double-blind technique. *N Engl J Med* 1959; 260:115–118.
4. Diamond EG, Kittle CF, Crockett JE: Comparison of internal mammary artery ligation and sham operation for angina pectoris. *Am J Cardiol* 1960; 5:483–486.
5. Favalaro RG: Saphenous vein graft in the surgical treatment of coronary artery disease. *J Thorac Cardiovasc Surg* 1969; 58:178–185.
6. Sheldon WC, Rincon G, Effler DB, et al: Vein graft surgery for coronary artery disease: Survival and angiographic results in 1,000 patients. *Circulation* 1973; 48(suppl 3):184–189.
7. Takaro T, Hultgren HN, Lipton MJ: The VA Cooperative Randomized Study of surgery for coronary arterial occlusive disease: II. Subgroup with significant left main lesions. *Circulation* 1976; 54(suppl 3):107.
8. Murphy ML, Hultgren HN, Detre K, et al: Treatment of chronic stable angina: A preliminary report of survival data of the randomized Veterans Administration Cooperative Study. *N Engl J Med* 1977; 297:621–627.
9. Takaro T, Hultgren HN, Detre KM, et al: The VA Cooperative Study of Stable Angina: Current status. *Circulation* 1982; 65(suppl 2):60–67.
10. Veterans Administration Coronary Artery Bypass Surgery Cooperative Study Group: Eleven-year survival in the Veterans Administration randomized trial of coronary bypass surgery for stable angina. *N Engl J Med* 1984; 311:1333–1345.
11. European Coronary Surgery Study Group: Long-term results of prospective randomized study of coronary artery bypass surgery in stable angina pectoris. *Lancet* 1982; 2:1173–1180.
12. Coronary Artery Surgery Study Principal Investigators and Associates: Coronary Artery Surgery Study (CASS): A randomized trial of coronary artery bypass surgery: Survival data. *Circulation* 1983; 68:939–950.
13. Passamani E, Davis KB, Gillespie MJ, et al: A randomized trial of coronary artery bypass surgery: Survival of patients with a low ejection fraction. *N Engl J Med* 1985; 312:1665–1670.
14. European Coronary Surgery Study Group: Survival, myocardial infarction, and employment status in a prospective randomized study of coronary bypass surgery. *Circulation* 1985; 72(suppl 5):90–101.

15. DeRouen TA, Hammermeister KE, Dodge HT: Comparison of the effects on survival after coronary artery surgery in subgroups of patients from the Seattle Heart Watch. *Circulation* 1981; 63:537–545.
16. Hammermeister KE: The effect of coronary bypass surgery on survival. *Prog Cardiovasc Dis* 1983; 15:297–333.
17. DeRouen TA, Hammermeister KE, Zia M, et al: Comparisons of survival between medically and surgically treated patients in a nonrandomized study, in Hammermeister KE (ed): *Coronary Bypass Surgery: The Late Results*. New York, Praeger Publishers, 1983, pp 229–250.
18. Gersh BJ, Kronmal RA, Schaff HV, et al: Comparison of coronary artery bypass surgery and medical therapy in patients 65 years of age or older: A nonrandomized study from the Coronary Artery Surgery Study (CASS) registry. *N Engl J Med* 1985; 313:217–224.
19. Faxon DP, Myers WO, McCabe CH, et al: The influence of surgery on the natural history of angiographically documented left ventricular aneurysm: The Coronary Artery Surgery Study. *Circulation* 1986; 74:110–118.
20. Holmes DR Jr, Davis KB, Mock MB, et al: The effect of medical and surgical treatment on subsequent sudden cardiac death in patients with coronary artery disease: A report from the Coronary Artery Surgery Study. *Circulation* 1986; 73:1254–1263.
21. Hammermeister KE, DeRouen TA, Zia M, et al: Survival of medically treated coronary artery disease patients in the Seattle Heart Watch Angiography Registry, in Hammermeister KE (ed): *Coronary Bypass Surgery: The Late Results*. New York, Praeger Publishers, 1983, pp 167–194.

Negative
Thomas J. Ryan, M.D.

Within the carefully phrased statement that titles this debate there are clearly several distinct clinical questions that surface and warrant identification in the interest of meaningful discussion. It is hard to imagine that any sound clinician would naysay the benefits of CABG or PTCA in *all* patients with stable symptoms. Yet the seasoned clinician will be quick to suggest that there are indeed some patients with known CAD who need not undergo revascularization, by either CABG or PTCA, simply because they have demonstrable disease that is amenable to either procedure. In the real world of practice the question actually is "Should patients with stable symptoms undergo CABG or PTCA as a matter of routine?" To this I will answer with a firm no. There is ample evidence that a substantial number of patients with stable symptoms and known coronary disease have an excellent prognosis, and in them there is no evidence that revascularization procedures improve that favorable outcome.

Let us begin by defining the population about whom there may be some real debate, since patients with "stable symptoms" can be quite a heterogeneous group. That is to say, patients with severe symptoms (class III or IV in the Canadian Cardiovascular Society classification) can be both chronic and stable, i.e., have unchanging symptoms over periods of months, whose natural history and benefit from CABG differ greatly from those of patients with mild symptoms (class I and II) who are also chronic and stable. In the former group there is no issue. Revascularization has repeatedly shown greater benefit in the relief of symptoms than medical therapy. Of more importance in regard to patients with stable but severe symptoms, there is recent evidence from a large observational study using concurrent and matched controls that CABG significantly improves survival compared with medical therapy in severely symptomatic patients with three-vessel disease even in the face of normal ventricular function. In the same study, identical patients with less severe angina (class I and II) showed no benefit from surgical therapy if they had three-vessel disease and preserved ventricular function. This is an important consideration because it draws us back from a mindset that became established in the midsixties and early seventies. I refer to it as the "syllogism of the sixties," which reasons as follows: the number of vessels diseased predicts outcome, but the severity of angina does not predict the number of vessels diseased, therefore the severity of angina does not predict outcome. Though the flaw in this reasoning is readily obvious to the clinician who has treated patients with severe, intractable, or unstable angina, this same line of reasoning has led to an overemphasis on anatomy and underassessment of the importance of symptoms. All too often the patient with minimal symptoms is referred for revascularization on the basis of anatomy alone. Such a policy overlooks a large body of data that support *function* and *symptoms* as being of equal importance in determining prognosis for the patient with CAD.

To pursue the argument about patients with stable and *mild* symptoms, it is my premise that only those patients known to be at high risk should be considered for revascularization. Who are they? The majority have been identified for us in the populations composing the three large randomized trials, the VA Cooperative Study, the ECSS, and the CASS, which have addressed this question over the past 15 years. Though there are both explicit and implicit differences among the three trials, the findings after extended follow-up of the three populations are remarkably similar. Both the VA and ECSS found a significant advantage for surgical therapy in patients with left main coronary disease, patients with marked ST segment depression on an exercise electrocardiogram, or ST segment abnormalities on the resting electrocardiogram. None of the studies showed an advantage for surgical therapy in patients with single-vessel disease, and though ECSS found a benefit for all patients with three-vessel disease, CASS found a significant advantage only for patients with three-vessel disease and impaired ventricular function. In the most recent report on the survival of the CASS randomized population, the advantage for surgical assignment was confined to those patients with three-vessel disease and impaired ventricular function who demonstrated angina during an exercise treadmill test. Although the VA study is viewed by many as having been irreversibly flawed by an unacceptably high operative mortality (5%), the follow-up of this unique population has extended beyond 12 years and many important lessons continue to emerge. Retrospective analysis showed that survival was improved significantly in a high-risk tercile selected on the basis of New York Heart Association classification, history of myocardial infarction, history of hypertension, and resting ST segment abnormality on the electrocardiogram (Fig 1). This difference reached its maximum after 7 years of follow-up. However, between 7 and 11 years after surgery the rate of surgical mortality has accelerated, and at 11 years the two survival curves have converged. Since few internal mammary artery anastomoses were performed in the VA study, these observations suggest that the venous conduits are failing after about 7 years.

Data from the Montreal Heart Institute also indicate accelerated deterioration of vein grafts 5 to 7 years after surgery. The mean graft closure rate was 1% between 1 and 6 years after surgery but increased threefold or fourfold during the following 5 to 6 years. It is concluded that 75% of venous grafts are unsuitable 10 years after operation. The surgical experience at most major medical centers corroborates these findings, and the

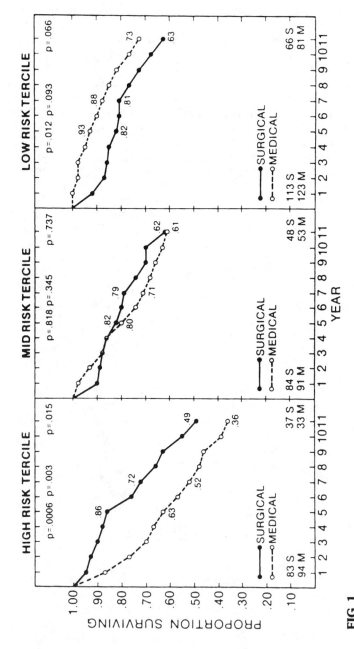

FIG 1.

Eleven-year cumulative survival rates for patients without left main coronary artery disease according to clinical risk. See text for definition of clinical risk. (From Bonow RO, Kent KM, Rosing DR, et al: Exercise-induced ischemia in mildly symptomatic patients with coronary artery disease and preserved left ventricular function: Identification of subgroups at risk of death during medical therapy. *N Engl J Med* 1984; 311:1333–1339. Reproduced by permission.)

majority of patients with CABG are requiring reoperation within 7 to 10 years. These facts suggest there is good reason to avoid premature bypass surgery. Revascularization accomplished by internal mammary conduits or by PTCA may not have the same limitation, but it is generally acknowledged that internal mammary conduits cannot provide complete revascularization in many instances, and the experience with PTCA, in addition to being limited, will always be influenced by progression of disease elsewhere in the same vessel.

Just as the randomized trials have identified subsets of patients with mild, stable symptoms who benefit from CABG, they also have identified patients who do not benefit from surgery. It is based on these patients that I take my stand that not all patients with stable symptoms should undergo CABG or PTCA. How well can they be identified? For the answer to this I am more influenced by a very recent publication from the CASS registry than I am by subset analyses of the comparatively small cohort that was randomized in CASS. One must remember that negative findings derived from comparatively small sample sizes are subject to a beta error and need to be interpreted with caution.

Weiner et al. analyzed the data from 5,303 nonrandomized patients from the CASS registry who underwent exercise testing and compared the results of bypass surgery with those of medical therapy alone over a period of 7 years' follow-up. When patients were grouped according to the amount of ST segment depression during exercise testing, those with less than 1 mm of ST segment depression had a slightly better 7-year survival rate with medical therapy (89% vs. 83%; P = .03), whereas among patients with 1 to 2 mm or greater ST segment depression, the 7-year survival rate was significantly higher in those treated surgically. The patients were then grouped according to the final exercise stage of the Bruce Protocol achieved. For those patients limited to stage I or less of exercise, surgery resulted in a slight survival advantage at 7 years (81% vs. 78%; P = .04), whereas for patients able to exercise into stage II or greater, survival rates were similar with medical and surgical therapy. The two individual exercise variables, ST segment response and final exercise stage achieved, were then combined into an exercise risk classification. The lower-risk subset comprised 1,545 patients without ischemic ST segment depression who could exercise to stage III or greater. The 7-year survival rates for the medical and surgical cohorts were virtually identical (91% vs. 90%; Fig 2). The higher-risk subset encompassed 789 patients who exhibited at least 1 mm of ST segment depression and who could exercise only into stage I or less. In contrast to the lower-risk subgroup, the 7-year survival rate for this subset was substantially improved with surgical compared with medical treatment (82% vs. 72%, respectively; P = .001).

The important point here is that these data are independent of angiographic data. The low-risk subset, those patients who showed less than 1

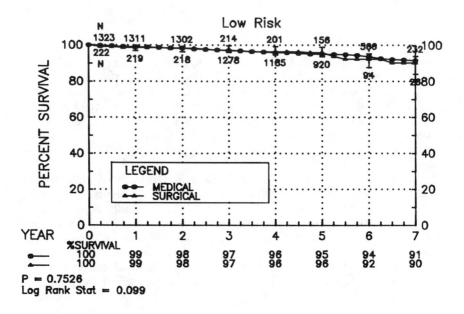

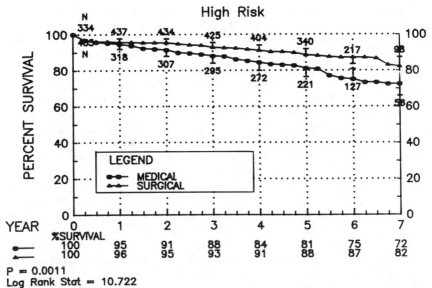

FIG 2.

Cumulative survival rates for the medical and surgical patients according to the exercise risk classification. A lower risk subgroup consisted of patients with less than 1 mm ST segment depression and a final exercise state of 3 mm or higher, whereas a higher risk subgroup consisted of patients with 1 mm or greater ST segment depression and a final exercise stage of 1 mm or less. (From *J Am Coll Cardiol* 1986; 741–748. Reproduced by permission.)

mm of ST segment depression and exercised into stage III or more of the Bruce Protocol, constituted 38% of the study population and had an annual mortality of 1.3%. It is to be recalled that this is the same as the annual mortality of the surgical patients in the randomized study. Since these 5,000 patients also had undergone coronary arteriography, it was possible to perform life table analyses stratifying for left ventricular function and extent of CAD. The results are interesting. For the 114 patients with one-vessel disease and for the 210 patients with two-vessel disease, 7-year survival rates were not different for those patients in the higher-risk exercise classification treated medically or surgically. Though the 398 patients with three-vessel disease in the higher-risk exercise classification showed a marked difference between the 7-year survival rates (81% for the surgical and 58% for the medical group; $P = .0001$), CABG did not improve survival in the lower-risk subset with three-vessel coronary disease. This rather simple classification into high and low risk by exercise testing thus seems helpful not only in identifying subsets of patients whose survival is enhanced by CABG but also in characterizing a subgroup of patients with excellent survival when treated medically.

Since patients with three-vessel CAD are not as readily and completely revascularized by PTCA as by surgery, this is the population with mild stable symptoms about which there seems to be the most clinical indecision regarding CABG. To some, this arises because of apparent discrepancies between the findings of the ECSS and the CASS studies. It was only those patients with impaired ventricular function and three-vessel disease that were found best treated by surgery in the CASS study. Those patients with three-vessel disease and normal ventricular function showed no advantage to surgical assignment compared with medical. In ECSS the population included only patients with normal ventricular function, yet, unlike the CASS population with normal ventricular function, there was a strong advantage for surgical therapy among those patients with three-vessel disease. This discrepancy is, I believe, readily explained by the "sicker population" in the European trial. It is to be noted that the annual mortality of the medically assigned patients in the European trial was 3.3% per year compared with 1.6% per year for the medically assigned patients in CASS. Furthermore, when reclassified according to the Canadian Cardiovascular Society classification, 42% of the ECSS population had class III symptoms, which, as we have pointed out, is a factor in survival. Lastly, another indication that the patients enrolled in the European study had more evidence of ischemia than the patients enrolled in CASS is to be found in a comparison of the exercise data obtained in the two populations. In the European trial, 89% of the population showed ST segment depression during exercise in contrast to 56% of the CASS population.

While I will acknowledge that quality of life as measured by exercise tolerance, diminution of symptoms, and the need for less medication is consistently better in patients who have undergone CABG, I believe we are discussing patients in whom this is not a substantive issue. When this question arises in my own practice, I have no hesitation in recommending surgery even for patients who have an excellent outlook with continued medical therapy. After all CABG, is a superb and safe operation. I do, however, keep in mind the risk-benefit ratio of CABG (Table 1).

Before concluding, it is worth noting that there is no evidence available that CABG prevents recurrent nonfatal myocardial infarction. All three randomized trials have failed to show any difference in the subsequent nonfatal myocardial infarction rates between patients randomized to medical or surgical therapy. Though this may have been an unexpected outcome when these studies were undertaken, in light of present knowledge that clearly demonstrates the role of thrombus formation in the pathogenesis of acute infarction, it is not so surprising that bypassing critical stenoses does not prevent thrombus formation from occurring at the site of lesser stenoses.

In conclusion, I would submit that there are substantial numbers of patients with mild, stable symptoms and three-vessel disease who do not require CABG. They are individuals who have normal ventricular function and show no evidence of ischemia during exercise testing. Since patients with single-vessel disease have an excellent survival, they are not candidates to undergo the risks of CABG. The same may be said for patients with two-vessel disease. However, both groups can safely undergo PTCA. Whether they should or not remains unproved, if the relief of symptoms is not the question at hand. If high-grade proximal stenoses are present in one or two vessels and significant ischemia is elicited by stress testing, I currently recommend PTCA. The role for this technique in patients with three-vessel disease will largely remain unanswered until the completion of the proposed NHLBI randomized trial.

TABLE 1.
Risk-Benefit of CABG

Operative mortality
Perioperative myocardial infarction
Cerebral dysfunction
Postcardiotomy syndrome
Wound infection
Hepatitis (AIDS?)
Progression of disease
Reoperation

Bibliography

1. Bonow RO, Kent KM, Rosing DR, et al: Exercise-induced ischemia in mildly symptomatic patients with coronary artery disease and preserved left ventricular function: Identification of subgroups at risk of death during medical therapy. *N Engl J Med* 1984; 311:1339.
2. Bourassa MG, Enjalbert M, Campeau L, et al: Progression of atherosclerosis in coronary arteries and bypass grafts: Ten years later. *Am J Cardiol* 1984; 53:102C–107C.
3. Coronary Artery Surgery Study Principal Investigators and Associates: Coronary Artery Surgery Study (CASS): A randomized trial of coronary artery bypass surgery: Quality of life in patients randomly assigned to treatment groups. *Circulation* 1983; 68:951–960.
4. Coronary Artery Surgery Study Principal Investigators and Associates: Coronary Artery Surgery Study (CASS): A randomized trial of coronary artery bypass surgery: Survival data. *Circulation* 1983; 68:939–950.
5. Coronary Artery Surgery Study Principal Investigators and Associates: Myocardial infarction and mortality in the Coronary Artery Surgery Study (CASS) randomized trial. *N Engl J Med* 1984; 310:750–758.
6. Detre KM, Takaro T, Hultgren H, et al: Long-term mortality and morbidity results of the Veterans Administration randomized trial of coronary artery bypass surgery. *Circulation* 1985; 72(suppl 5):84–89.
7. European Coronary Surgery Study Group: Long-term results of prospective randomised study of coronary artery bypass surgery in stable angina pectoris. *Lancet* 1982; 2:1173–1180.
8. European Coronary Surgery Study Group: Survival, myocardial infarction, and employment status in a prospective randomized study of coronary bypass surgery. *Circulation* 1985; 72(suppl 5):90–101.
9. Kaiser GC, Davis KB, Fisher LD, et al: Survival following coronary artery bypass grafting in patients with severe angina pectoris (CASS). *J Thorac Cardiovasc Surg* 1985; 89:513–524.
10. Killip T, Passamani E, Davis K, et al: Coronary Artery Surgery Study (CASS): A randomized trial of coronary bypass surgery: Eight years follow-up and survival in patients with reduced ejection fraction. *Circulation* 1985; 72(suppl 5):102–109.
11. Killip T, Ryan TJ: Randomized trials in coronary bypass surgery. *Circulation* 1985; 71:418–421.
12. Ryan TJ, Weiner DA, McCabe CH, et al: Exercise testing in the coronary artery surgery study randomized population. *Circulation* 1985; 72(suppl 5):31–38.
13. Takaro T, Hultgren H, Lipton M, et al: VA Cooperative Randomized Study for coronary arterial occlusive disease: II. Left main disease. *Circulation* 1976; 54(suppl 3):107–117.
14. Veterans Administration Coronary Artery Bypass Surgery Cooperative Study Group: Eleven-year survival in the Veterans Administration randomized trial of coronary bypass surgery for stable angina. *N Engl J Med* 1984; 311:1333–1345.

Rebuttal: Affirmative

Karl E. Hammermeister, M.D.

My opponent has presented several convincing arguments backed with solid data (much of it from the CASS, with which he has been actively involved) that many patients with stable symptoms do not require a revascularization procedure, be it PTCA or CABG. I have tried to present arguments on the opposite side of the issue, that some of these patients will benefit from a revascularization procedure. Despite our assigned positions on opposite sides of the question, we agree in many instances. I suspect that if we were both asked to evaluate the same ten patients with stable symptoms, we should make the same general recommendation (medical therapy vs. revascularization) in seven or eight of the ten. This would include the need for revascularization in patients with left main CAD and in patients with three-vessel disease and left ventricular dysfunction. We would also recommend medical therapy in patients with mild, stable symptoms who have only single-vessel disease or two-vessel disease not involving the left anterior descending coronary artery.

We both point out the conflict between the ECSS and the CASS performed in the United States and Canada in regard to patients with three-vessel disease and normal left ventricular function. Dr. Ryan uses the recently published study by Weiner, himself, and others[1] to assist in resolving this conflict: patients with three-vessel disease who exhibit ischemic ST segment depression and markedly impaired exercise capacity on exercise testing appear to experience substantial survival benefit from revascularization. Again, I agree and note that these results are similar to those published earlier by us from the Seattle Heart Watch.[2]

This brings me to my major point in this rebuttal statement: the seeming paradox between the importance of the medical history and its unreliability. The presence and severity of ischemic myocardial symptoms are central to the therapeutic scheme proposed by the opposing essay: patients with few or no symptoms do not require revascularization unless they have left ventricular dysfunction and three-vessel disease. First, let me affirm my conviction that the medical history contains 70% to 80% of the diagnostic information available to us in the evaluation of patients with possible coronary heart disease, as beautifully documented in the now classic study by Weiner and colleagues.[3] At the same time, I must express my alarm that history taking appears to be a lost art for all too many of our medical students, house staff, and even some of my faculty colleagues.

Despite the vital importance of the medical history, particularly in arriving at a diagnosis, it seems to me too subjective and nonreproducible to serve as the primary source on which to base a decision as important as the undertaking of a revascularization procedure. It is well documented that there is a poor correlation between symptoms as reflected in the New York Heart Association functional classification and functional capacity as measured by a symptom-limited exercise test.[4] There are many reasons for this, only one of which is my lament over the loss of and failure to teach and learn history-taking skills. The medical history is highly dependent on the patient's and physician's personalities and the interaction between the two. Some patients are by nature stoic and do not or cannot reveal the full nature of their symptoms. Some patients are so anxious and hypochondriacal that it becomes very difficult to sort out symptoms due to myocardial ischemia from psychosomatic symptoms. Some patients, perhaps most at one time or another, have no symptoms with myocardial ischemia. We are just beginning to study the prevalence of silent ischemia and the characteristics of patients who experience it. However, we have virtually no knowledge of its prognostic significance or how it should influence the indications for revascularization.

Given the limitations of historical information, it seems to me that a wider database together with considerable flexibility and clinical judgment have to be exercised in regard to recommending revascularization. The arrival at such a recommendation requires a truly "multivariate equation," which must involve, in addition to symptoms, coronary anatomy, and left ventricular function, the mass of myocardium placed at jeopardy by proximal stenoses, the quality of the vessels for the revascularization procedure proposed, the general medical status of the patient, the patient's age, the risk of the revascularization procedure, diabetes, continued cigarette smoking, left ventricular hypertrophy, peripheral vascular disease, chronic obstructive pulmonary disease, and the patient's desire. Some have overinterpreted the results of the CASS to mean that patients with CAD with few or no symptoms and good left ventricular function have a good prognosis and require little further evaluation. I believe that there are substantial numbers of patients within this large subgroup who will be at increased risk for cardiac death and will benefit from revascularization. Dr. Ryan has emphasized that marked exercise intolerance and ST segment depression during exercise identify patients whose survival is prolonged with revascularization. Other characteristics that point toward improved survival with revascularization are absence of congestive heart failure, absence of cardiomegaly, absence of diabetes, ST segment depression on the resting electrocardiogram, impaired pressure-rate product at maximal exercise, and absence of peripheral vascular disease.[5]

To summarize, there is general agreement that for patients with CAD with stable, mild, or no symptoms, those with left main coronary artery obstruction or those with three-vessel disease with left ventricular systolic dysfunction generally have improved survival with revascularization and should be offered the procedure. However, even in this group there will be some who will not experience survival benefit because of high operative risk due to age, general medical condition, or severe left ventricular dysfunction, or when complete revascularization is not achievable because of distal vessel disease. There is also agreement that revascularization does not prolong survival in patients with limited CAD, such as single-vessel disease or two-vessel disease not involving the left anterior descending coronary artery.

On the other hand, I have argued that presence or absence of symptoms is a sufficiently unreliable measure of risk (particularly when some patients appear to have defective perception of myocardial ischemia) to be relied on as the major criterion of intervention. The mass of viable myocardium distal to severe coronary artery stenosis, ST segment depression on the resting electrocardiogram, exercise intolerance, and exercise-induced ischemia all need to be considered.

References

1. Weiner DA, Ryan TJ, McCabe CH, et al: The role of exercise testing in identifying patients with improved survival after coronary artery bypass surgery. *J Am Coll Cardiol* 1986; 8:741–748.
2. Bruce RA, DeRouen TA, Hammermeister KE: Noninvasive screening criteria for enhanced 4-year survival after aortocoronary bypass surgery. *Circulation* 1979; 60:638–646.
3. Weiner DA, Ryan TJ, McCabe CH, et al: Exercise stress testing: Correlations among history of angina, ST-segment response and prevalence of coronary-artery disease in the Coronary Artery Surgery Study (CASS). *N Engl J Med* 1979; 301:230–235.
4. Goldman L, Hashimoto B, Cook EF, et al: Comparative reproducibility and validity of systems for assessing cardiovascular functional class: Advantages of a new specific activity scale. *Circulation* 1981; 64:1227–1234.
5. DeRouen TA, Hammermeister KE, Dodge HT: Comparison of the effects on survival after coronary artery surgery in subgroups of patients from the Seattle Heart Watch. *Circulation* 1981; 63:537–545.

Rebuttal: Negative
Thomas J. Ryan, M.D.

There is much to agree with in Dr. Hammermeister's position paper, and it should be obvious from the outset that we concur on the substantive issue that CABG has been demonstrated to prolong life *in some patients,* wholly apart from its demonstrated superiority in relieving anginal symptoms when compared with medical treatment for patients with symptomatic CAD. Logically, these are the patients who should undergo CABG or PTCA, even in the face of stable symptoms. The corollary to this statement, that there are some patients whose prognosis is so good that improved survival will not be seen with any form of therapy short of the "fountain of youth," is the issue I would argue further.

Dr. Hammermeister and his group have made notable contributions to the medical vs. surgical debate relating to patients with CAD from their observational data taken from the nonrandomized Seattle Heart Watch Coronary Arteriography Registry. Understandably, this experience has shaped much of his view, which I conclude is rather pro-surgery and, in some measure, explains his preference for the data derived from the ECSS randomized trial rather than the CASS trial. Although he acknowledges that "it is now widely recognized that selection bias . . . strongly influences the outcome of nonrandomized studies," Dr. Hammermeister maintains that multivariate statistical techniques allow appropriate adjustment for baseline differences between medically and surgically treated patients. Although such analysis does not carry the scientific strength of a randomized trial, he maintains the population studied is more likely to be representative of the "real world" because there is much less selectivity than occurs with entry of patients into a randomized trial. Though this may be true, all observational studies must be interpreted with caution, even when sophisticated multivariate statistical techniques are used to adjust for baseline differences between medically and surgically treated patients because such adjustments are, at best, imperfect. Obviously, not all the considerations that enter into the bedside decision that determines whether a patient is treated medically or surgically are captured or entered as measurable variables in the statistical model. The Seattle Heart Watch data give testimony to some of the peculiar conclusions that can be drawn. That data bank suggests that surgery improves survival in patients without cardiomegaly but not in those with; in patients without a history of congestive heart failure but not in those with; in patients without peripheral vascular disease but not in those with. These findings seem to fly in the face of data derived from the more rigorous randomized approach used in both the European and CASS trials.

An additional note of caution should be directed at comparisons between a group of patients receiving a specific therapy and age-matched controls taken from the general population. Certainly, patients undergoing coronary arteriography for consideration of surgery do not include patients who have terminal renal disease, lymphoma, or malignant neoplasms that are included in general population statistics.

Other than these caveats, I will go on record as a proponent of observational studies derived from large data banks that have been appropriately analyzed and whose conclusions are tempered by the recognition that any differences found between populations could be explained by unmeasured variables. Certainly, it is my belief that the greatest contributions to be derived from CASS are its many registry studies that rely totally on observational analysis.

Dr. Hammermeister argues that randomized trials "may present too conservative a viewpoint, primarily because the patients selected are not representative of the general population of patients with coronary heart disease being considered for coronary bypass surgery." He then gravitates to the data derived from the European trial, claiming that "it seems likely that the majority of patients in this study may have had mild angina," yet he views the study as being markedly different in outcome from the CASS trial. I have gone to some length to point out the evidence that the European population was generally more ill with their coronary disease, as indicated by an annual mortality of 3.3% per year for those medically assigned; 42% of the European population had class III symptoms and 89% of the population showed ST segment depression during exercise, compared with only 56% of the CASS population. This is true even when the European population is analyzed according to a 75% stenosis as a definition of significant coronary disease, although the original analysis was done using a 50% stenosis. These data confirm what most contemporary cardiologists already know, i.e., the sicker the patient, the greater their need for revascularization, all else being equal. Germane to this debate, however, is the identification of patients who do not require revascularization. In this regard, the CASS trial seems to make the greatest contribution. To dismiss it as a study that "in some way selected an extremely low-risk group of patients" and is flawed because the randomized population constitutes only 3% of the patients then undergoing coronary arteriography for suspected CAD is to fail to understand the question being posed.

The CASS was designed in the midseventies, after bypass surgery was well established as a major surgical procedure that could be performed with a low risk and resulted in angina relief in most patients. It was reasoned that a revascularization procedure, which was successful in alleviating bothersome symptoms, might also extend life or prevent recurrent myocardial infarctions in those known to have significant obstructing coronary lesions but who had minimal or virtually no symptoms of angina. The CASS was thus formulated around the question of whether survival could be enhanced in individuals with potentially lethal coronary lesions but mild to moderate symptoms. Fundamentally, the question was to what degree should the indications for bypass surgery *be expanded*. What, for example, should be the approach to asymptomatic survivors of a myocardial infarction? Conservative estimates would place this number at about 200,000 patients per year. Doubling this number might approximate the additional population with CAD and mild symptoms. If revascularization surgery was to be extended to this category (and number) of patients on the ground that it prolonged life, the evidence would have to be compelling. Rigorous testing applied to the specific population in question, using a prospective randomized control study design, was acknowledged as the most stringent means of answering this important question that harbored both medical and economic implications.

Actually, the 780 randomized patients (the numerator) composed 37.2% of the study population, i.e., those judged suitable for randomization. Unlike any of the other large randomized trials, the CASS investigators have provided a clear and important follow-up of the remaining 1,315 patients (the denominator), who, although qualified for randomization, were assigned therapy by physician preference.[1] It has been claimed that the majority of patients in the randomized trial were considered by clinical judgment not to be surgical candidates.[2] It is true that CASS was designed to test the hypothesis that surgery would prolong life in patients who do not require surgical palliation of severe symptoms. It is thus understandable that the CASS registry, which included all patients undergoing coronary arteriography at the time, included a much larger subset for whom the decision had already been made.

To underscore the validity of the randomized population as being representative of the true study population (all those qualifying for randomization, i.e., randomizable), baseline characteristics for the two populations were similar. Table 2 shows that there was a proportional distribution of angiographic severity of disease between the 780 randomized patients and the 1,315 randomizable patients who were followed up. On the other hand, physician bias is evident in the form of therapy selected for the randomizable population, as illustrated in Table 3. By study design, the distribution of one-, two-, or three-vessel disease was similar in the randomized cohort between medical and surgical groups. In the randomizable patients who received therapy according to physician decision, it can be seen that the majority of patients with single-vessel disease received medical therapy, whereas the majority of patients with three-vessel disease received surgical therapy. Though this reflected clinical thinking at the time and was largely influenced by the already published results of the European trial, it is important to note that subsequent survival curves for the two populations were virtually identical, whether they received medical or surgical therapy.

To me, this constitutes compelling evidence that the lessons learned from the CASS randomized study population are applicable to the popu-

TABLE 2.
Preservation of Proportionality*†

No. of Diseased Vessels (≥70% Narrowing)	Randomized (n = 780)	Randomizable (n = 1,315)
1	27.4	31.8
2	39.5	35.2
3	33.1	33.0
Proximal LAD	31.5	33.5

*From Coronary Artery Surgery Study Principal Investigators and Associates: Coronary Artery Surgery Study (CASS): A randomized trial of coronary artery bypass surgery: Comparability of entry characteristics and survival in randomized patients and non-randomized patients meeting randomization criteria. *J Am Coll Cardiol* 1984; 3:114–128. Reproduced by permission.
†Values are percentages. LAD indicates left anterior descending coronary artery. No difference was significant.

TABLE 3.
Baseline Inequities: Angiographic Data*†

No. of Diseased Vessels (≥70% Narrowing)	Randomized		Nonrandomized	
	Medicine (n = 390)	Surgery (n = 390)	Medicine (n = 745)	Surgery (n = 570)
1	27.4	27.4	40.3	20.7†
2	38.0	41.0	36.8	33.2
3	34.6	31.5	23.0	46.1†
Proximal LAD	30.3	32.8	27.4	46.1†

*From Coronary Artery Surgery Study Principal Investigators and Associates: Coronary Artery Surgery Study (CASS): A randomized trial of coronary artery bypass surgery: Comparability of entry characteristics and survival in randomized patients and non-randomized patients meeting randomization criteria. *J Am Coll Cardiol* 1984; 3:114–128. Reproduced by permission.
†Values are percentages. LAD indicates left anterior descending coronary artery. $P < .001$.

lation at large who are mildly symptomatic with angiographically proved coronary disease. The study has served me well as a clinician in identifying those patients with stable symptoms who do not, for the moment, seem to require CABG or PTCA.

References

1. Coronary Artery Surgery Study Principal Investigators and Associates: Coronary Artery Surgery Study (CASS): A randomized trial of coronary artery bypass surgery: Comparability of entry characteristics and survival in randomized patients and non-randomized patients meeting randomization criteria. *J Am Coll Cardiol* 1984; 3:114–128.
2. Gunnar RM, Loeb HS: An alternative interpretation of the CASS study. *Circulation* 1985; 71:193–194.

This debate illustrates the point that polar views on this important topic have become less divergent with time. The positions taken by the two debators are not strikingly dissimilar. Both argue persuasively for a thoughtful selection of patients for CABG when intolerable symptoms are not an indication. Most cardiologists would agree that for the symptomatic patient or the patient who cannot tolerate medication, bypass or angioplasty when feasible are excellent therapies, producing a major improvement in lifestyle. The debatable topic continues to be when to recommend these therapies for patients whose symptoms are not severe or disabling with or without medication. Angioplasty is now performed widely, but there are no data available on the influence of this procedure on prognosis, so that it is employed for relief of symptoms or when there is an intuition that prognosis might be improved. The use of surgery is a bigger question because the risks, discomfort, and expense to the patient are greater, and there is now understanding that this is indeed a palliative, not curative, procedure with a finite life span. Second and third operations are now quite common, but results clearly decline with each surgical procedure. Hence, the timing of surgery for the patient with a long-standing chronic disease becomes a paramount question. There are still physicians who recommend CABG whenever the anatomic situation is favorable, but they seem to be increasingly in the minority. The balanced view presented by both authors in this debate seems to be prevailing.

Both Drs. Hammermeister and Ryan emphasize the importance of the history in deciding on when to recommend an operation. Both understand that ischemic heart disease with more severe symptoms indicates a more grave prognosis than when the symptoms are not severe. Treadmill testing is an important adjunct to the history, providing objective information to support or deny the historical findings, with poor exercise capacity with evidence of severe ischemia by electrocardiography indicating a poor prognosis. Both agree that patients with left main CAD or three-vessel disease and abnormal ventricular function may show improved survival as a result of surgery, if the anatomic situation is suitable for an operation, and that surgery does not influence prognosis in single-vessel disease or in some patients with two-vessel involvement. The major divergence of the two is in the patient with three-vessel disease and normal ventricular function or two-vessel disease with anterior descending involvement. In these settings, Dr. Hammermeister would favor a surgical approach, whereas Dr. Ryan would use medical therapy unless there were strong indication of severe ischemia by history or treadmill testing. Here Dr. Hammermeister is more strongly influenced by the results of ECSS and his own data from Seattle, and Dr. Ryan relies more heavily on the results of the CASS study. Each author presents an excellent defense of his position, and it is up to the reader to decide which approach he or she would favor based on the evidence presented. I tend to agree with Dr. Ryan's position and believe that the CASS data are an important resource to utilize in dealing with patients with mild symptoms. Dr. Hammermeister makes the excellent point that such decisions are highly individual and require a strong consideration of the amount of myocardium supplied by obstructed arteries that is at risk for ischemia or permanent injury.

Coronary bypass surgery has had an immense influence on the practice of cardiovascular medicine. As with all therapies, the initial overenthusiastic application has been tempered by more sober analysis of the efficacy of the procedure with time and the accumulation of objective data regarding long-term benefits. This has allowed a more rational utilization of the procedure. Discussions such as this debate highlight this point.

Mild Hypertension Should Be Managed With Drug Therapy

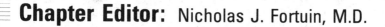

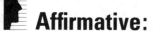

Chapter Editor: Nicholas J. Fortuin, M.D.

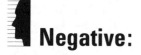

Affirmative:

Marvin Moser, M.D.
Clinical Professor of Medicine, Department
of Internal Medicine, Yale University School
of Medicine, New Haven, Connecticut

Negative:

Norman M. Kaplan, M.D.
Professor of Internal Medicine, Chief,
Hypertension Division, Department of
Internal Medicine, University of Texas
Southwestern Medical School, Dallas, Texas

Debates in Medicine 1:30–63, 1988
© 1988, Year Book Medical Publishers, Inc.
0887-218X/88/01-030-063-$04.00

Affirmative
Marvin Moser, M.D.

Most physicians would agree with the available epidemiologic data on hypertension that indicate an increased risk for cardiovascular disease if blood pressures remain at levels of 140/90 mm Hg or higher. Most would also agree that patients with diastolic blood pressures (DBPs) of 100 mm Hg or more will benefit from a reduction of blood pressure by pharmacologic therapy. There is a difference of opinion, however, regarding the effects of treatment on cardiovascular complications in patients with mild hypertension, i.e., those with DBPs between 90 and 100 mm Hg. Many investigators believe that the evidence suggesting benefit from treatment is not firm enough to make general recommendations for treatment, especially if management involves the use of medication. A major argument against treatment of patients with mild hypertension is that "many must be treated to benefit a few" and that the adverse reactions of specific therapies may be frequent or serious enough in many patients to cancel out the possible benefits of therapy.

I disagree with this opinion and believe that mild hypertension should be treated pharmacologically if, after a suitable period of nonpharmacologic treatment, blood pressures have not been reduced to levels below 140/90 mm Hg. Data indicate that the benefit of treatment outweighs the risk and that blood pressure can be lowered with relatively few adverse reactions or metabolic changes in most patients and with little effect on life-style. Although the ideal pharmacologic approach to the lowering of blood pressure has not been found and indeed may be years away from discovery, present medications, if used appropriately, will lower blood pressures to normal levels in approximately 90% of patients, with a reduction of morbidity and mortality.

Resistance among some investigators to treat the mildly hypertensive patient is also based on what I believe to be a narrow interpretation of the major clinical trials. The following arguments and data justify a pharmacologic approach to therapy if blood pressures remain above 140/90 mm Hg. If the following precautions are taken before the institution of pharmacologic management, the number of patients who may be treated unnecessarily can be reduced to a minimum.

1. A persistent elevation of blood pressure should be verified. In the major clinical trials, especially the Medical Research Council (MRC) and Australian trials, approximately 20% of patients who were initially randomized as hypertensive, with DBPs over 95 mm Hg, had a decrease in DBPs to levels of 90 mm Hg or below. This normalization usually occurred within 3 to 4 months. Blood pressures should be rechecked, therefore, on at least two occasions over a 3- to 4-month period before beginning ther-

apy. If pressure decreases to under 140/90 mm Hg, the patient should then be followed up at 6-month intervals. This will immediately reduce the potential number of patients to be treated by about 20%.

2. During this initial 3- to 4-month period of observation, various non-pharmacologic methods of management should be tried. Our own results with these techniques have not been as good as reported by some investigators. If, however, the patient is able to reduce weight (if appropriate) and sodium intake to approximately 80 to 85 mEq/day, to go on a modified exercise program, and to decrease alcohol intake (if it is more than 3 or 4 oz/day), it is conceivable that another 15% to 20% of patients will become normotensive. These patients should also be followed up at 6-month intervals and treated only if their DBPs return to levels of 90 mm Hg or more.

The Clinical Trials

We must then look to the clinical trials to find answers to the question of what to do with patients whose DBPs remain between 90 and 100 mm Hg.

Most of the clinical trials used end points of fatal or nonfatal strokes, fatal or nonfatal coronary occlusions, or specific cardiovascular events such as dissecting aneurysms, etc., to calculate statistical benefit of treatment. These are the data that most physicians have used to determine whether or not treatment is justified. The comparative data on progression from mild to severe hypertension in treated and untreated patients should, however, also be considered in making this judgment. These are usually ignored in evaluating the benefits of the treatment of patients with less severe disease.

In the five major clinical trials, which employed placebos or untreated controls, i.e., the U.S. Public Health Service Study, The Veterans Administration Cooperative Study, the Australian Trial, the Oslo Study, and the MRC Study, a total of 1,318 of 11,129 subjects progressed to severe hypertension, with DBPs in excess of 110 to 130 mm Hg in the placebo or control groups. In the active-treatment groups, only 82 of 11,206 progressed (Table 1). The lack of progression in treated patients suggests an important indication for early therapy.

Other factors are often ignored in evaluating clinical trials and the possible benefits of treatment of mild hypertension. There are no data available, for example, to answer the question of "undetectable vascular changes" that may have occurred in the course of these short-term (3- to 7-year) trials in patients whose blood pressures remained elevated. If physicians agree that prolonged hypertension increases the progression of atherosclerotic changes in blood vessel walls, presumably by damaging the endothelium and increasing cholesterol turnover, then it is possible that by

TABLE 1.
Effect of Treatment on Preventing Progression From Mild to More Severe Hypertension: Findings From Major Clinical Trials*

| | No. of Patients | | | |
| | Placebo | | Active Treatment | |
Study (Range for Mild Hypertension, mm Hg)	Mild Hypertension	Progressed to More Severe	Mild Hypertension	Progressed to More Severe
USPHS (90–114)	196	24†	193	0
VA Cooperative (90–114)	194	20	186	0
Australian (95–109)	1,706	198	1,721	5
Oslo (90–110)‡	379	65	406	1
MRC (90–109)	8,654	1,011	8,700	76
Total	11,129	1,318	11,206	82

*USPHS indicates U.S. Public Health Service Study.
†DBP > 130 mm Hg.
‡12.5% of patients had systolic hypertension only.

keeping patients at normotensive levels, this type of undetectable change may be prevented—perhaps another argument for early treatment (which, as yet, cannot be proved in humans).

Results from the clinical trials indicate that though blood pressure lowering may be beneficial, even after organ damage has occurred, complications are fewer if therapy is instituted before the development of target organ involvement. For example, in the Hypertension Detection and Follow-up Program (HDFP) study (Table 2), patients without pretreatment target organ damage experienced a 4.5% death rate in stepped care (SC) vs. a 5.8% death rate in referred care (RC), a definite benefit in the SC, or more vigorously treated, group of patients. There was also a significant reduction in deaths in the SC compared with the RC patients when pretreatment target organ damage was present (15.6% vs. 20%), but a much higher overall mortality in both groups.

These are important facts to consider when making a decision of when and how to treat mild hypertension. I do not believe that we should wait for evidence of arteriolar involvement in the retina, the presence of left ventricular hypertrophy, or persistent elevations of DBPs to 100 mm Hg or above before considering specific therapy.

The "U.S. Experience"

Although anecdotal, "nonrandomized or uncontrolled" experiences are not often accepted by the scientific community, the experience in the United States is of interest with regard to the course of hypertensive disease over the past 20 to 30 years. In the 1940s and 1950s, it was common to observe hospitalized patients with congestive heart failure secondary to hypertensive heart disease; accelerated or malignant hypertension, renal failure secondary to hypertension, and strokes of hypertensive origin were common. Over the past 20 to 30 years in the United States, the occurrence of accelerated or malignant hypertension, pulmonary edema secondary to hypertension, and/or strokes has decreased dramatically. Although this trend cannot be attributed solely to the early treatment of hypertension, it is a fact that should be considered by those who suggest withholding therapy in less severely hypertensive subjects. In countries other than the United States, where a vigorous approach has not been taken, the incidence of hypertensive complications has decreased at a slower rate; in the United States the stroke death rate alone has dropped by over 50% in the past 15 years, a record unmatched by any of the industrialized countries. Some of this decrease may be secondary to a decrease in smoking and a change in eating or exercise habits, but a large degree of success in this area must be attributed to the early treatment of hypertension.

What do the clinical trials tell us about the treatment of less severe de-

TABLE 2.
HDPF: Percentage Reduction in Mortality in Stratum 1 Subjects According to Presence or Absence of Pretreatment Target-Organ Damage*

Target Organ Damage	Stepped Care (SC)		Referred Care (RC)		Reduction in Mortality (SC:RC), %
	Sample Size	No. of Deaths (Rate, %)	Sample Size	No. of Deaths (Rate, %)	
Present	501	78 (15.6)	460	92 (20)	22.0
Absent	3,402	153 (4.5)	3,462	199 (5.7)	22.4

*Stratum 1 subjects had DBP of 90 to 104 mm Hg. Target organ damage included left ventricular hypertrophy on electrocardiogram, history of myocardial infarction, stroke, intermittent claudication, and serum creatinine level over 1.7 mg/dl.

grees of hypertension? In examining data that are available from the clinical trials on approximately 44,000 patients, it is apparent that not only were complications from strokes, fatal and nonfatal, and overall cardiovascular events decreased, but there was a trend, although not statistically significant in some trials, toward a reduction in coronary events. The recently completed European Working Party Study in Hypertension in the Elderly (EWPHE) and the HDFP study reported a significant reduction in deaths from coronary artery disease in specially treated patients.

The HDFP study in the United States has answered some of the questions left unanswered by the Veterans Administration and Public Health Service clinical trials. This study involved over 10,900 men and women recruited by population-based screening of over 158,000 people, aged 30 to 69 years, in 14 communities. The hypertensive patients were randomly divided into two equal groups. Over 70% of the patients in each group were classified as having mild hypertension (DBP, 90 to 104 mm Hg).

Group 1, or the RC group, received customary or routine care that was available in the community. Group 2, or the SC group, was treated in special hypertension centers that utilized the SC method of treatment as originally advocated in the First Joint National Committee Report in the United States. This included the use of a diuretic as step 1 therapy. Potassium-sparing agents were used as supplementary therapy where necessary. Reserpine (0.1 to 0.25 mg/day) was the preferred step 2 drug and was used in over 40% of patients, with methyldopa (500 to 2,000 mg/day) used as an alternative medication. The addition of a vasodilator, hydralazine (step 3), or a step 4 drug, such as guanethidine, was necessary in some cases.

Mildly hypertensive patients (DBP, 90 to 104 mm Hg) in both the SC and the RC groups demonstrated a decrease in both systolic blood pressure and DBP over the 5-year period of the trial. Blood pressures decreased from 153/96 to 129/83 mm Hg in the SC group compared with a decrease from 153/96 to 141/88 mm Hg in the RC group.

By the fifth year, approximately 65% of the SC patients with mild hypertension had achieved goal blood pressure, defined as a DBP of 90 mm Hg or less or a decrease of at least 10 mm Hg in DBP if the initial pressures were under 100 mm Hg. Approximately 45% of the RC patients had also achieved goal blood pressure.

All-cause mortality in patients with mild hypertension was 20% lower in the SC group. Forty-five percent fewer deaths from strokes and 20% fewer deaths from coronary heart disease were noted in the SC group. The incidence of angina and myocardial infarctions was also decreased in the SC group. However, statistically significant differences in mortality were not noted in patients below 50 years of age (this finding was expected, given the mild degree of the hypertension and the short duration of the study). Cardiovascular mortality in white women was similar in both the RC and the SC groups, reflecting the high degree of compliance of this subset of patients in the RC group and the fact that blood pressure differences were less in white women than in the entire cohort when the SC group was compared with the RC group.

Mortality decreased for patients at all levels of initial DBP, even at pressures under 100 mm Hg. Of great importance is the fact that mortality was significantly reduced in the subjects with pretreatment DBPs of 90 to 94 mm Hg, as well as in patients with DBPs between 95 and 99 mm Hg (Table 3). In considering the results of this trial, it is important to remember that both groups were treated. As experience from previous trials has shown, differences would probably have been greater if a nontreated or placebo control group had been part of the study. Mortality was greatly increased in both groups of patients who had pretreatment end-organ damage—a strong argument for early treatment.

Some of the critics of the HDFP study point out that blood pressure lowering may not have been the only reason for a decrease in mortality, since both cardiovascular and noncardiovascular mortality was reduced in the SC group. Could the reduced mortality have been the result of better overall medical care? This is possible, but it appears that the blood pressure differences accounted for the differences in outcome; systolic pressure and DBP were consistently higher in both the RC and SC patients who subsequently died compared with levels in survivors, regardless of the type of care they received. In addition, there were no significant differences in cholesterol levels, weight changes, or smoking habits in the two groups to account for the difference in overall mortality. The reversal of left ventricular hypertrophy and reduction in strokes and stroke deaths in a higher percentage of SC than RC patients are findings that are difficult to explain as a result of "better general medical care." The HDFP study results ap-

TABLE 3.
HDFP Study: Five-Year Mortality Rates,
Stratum I

Pretreatment DBP, mm Hg	Rate per 100 Participants		Reduction in Mortality for SC Patients, %
	SC	RC	
90–104	5.9	7.4	20.3
90–94	5.7	7.3	21.9
95–99	5.0	6.5	23.1
100–104	7.5	8.7	13.8

pear to indicate that it was the greater degree of blood pressure lowering that made the difference.

The Australian Therapeutic Trial in Mild Hypertension involved over 3,000 men and women and compared a treatment group with a placebo group. Overall cardiovascular deaths were reduced by 70%, and cerebrovascular events, both fatal and nonfatal, were reduced by 50% in the treated group. The number of deaths in both the placebo and treatment groups was small, as might be expected in a short-term trial in an all-white population with mild hypertension (Tables 4 and 5). The reduction of ischemic heart disease events in the treatment group was not statistically significant, although there was a downward trend (70 events in the active treatment group vs. 88 in the placebo group). Benefit was noted in patients with initial DBPs over 95 mm Hg. (Patients with pretreatment DBPs under 95 mm Hg were not included in the study.)

The higher rate of complications in the placebo group was consistent with the fact that only 25% of this group achieved average blood pressure levels of 90 mm Hg or below, compared with 65% in the actively treated group; 20% of placebo-treated patients had average DBPs over 100 mm Hg compared with only 5% in the active-treatment group. Diastolic blood pressures rose to levels over 100 mm Hg in 198 (12%) of the 1,706 patients in the placebo group.

TABLE 4.
Australian Therapeutic Trial: Incidence of Fatal and Nonfatal TEPs in Patients With Mild Hypertension*

TEPs	Active Treatment (n = 1,721)		Placebo (n = 1,706)	
	No. of TEPs	Rate	No. of TEPs	Rate
Fatal				
Cardiovascular	4	0.8	13	2.5†
Noncardiovascular	5	0.9	6	1.2
Total	9	1.7	19	3.7‡
Nonfatal	82	15.5	108	20.8†
All TEPs	91	17.2	127	24.5‡

*TEPs indicates trial end points. Rates are rate per 1,000 person-years of exposure to risk.
†$P < .05$.
‡$P < .025$.
§$P < .01$.

TABLE 5.
Deaths in Patients With Mild to Moderate Hypertension: Findings From Several Clinical Trials Compared With Australian Trial

Study	Deaths From Cerebrovascular Disease, %			Deaths From Coronary Heart Disease, %		
	Untreated Group	Treated Group	Difference, %	Untreated Groups	Treated Group	Difference, %
VA	10.3	2.7	−74	5.7	3.2	−44
Australian	0.35	0.17	−50	0.6	0.3	−50
HDFP	0.9	0.5	−44	2.7	2.2	−19

The Oslo study involved over 800 patients with mild hypertension who were treated over a 5-year period. This study failed to demonstrate a significant decrease in total cardiovascular events in the treated group, but the results did indicate a decrease in deaths from cerebrovascular accidents. Of the 395 patients in the control group (who did not receive placebo), 65 (16%) were placed in the treatment group when their blood pressures rose above 180/110 mm Hg, at which point it was deemed unethical to withhold treatment.

Because the number of persons studied and the number of complications and deaths were small, the results of this study probably cannot be compared with those of other studies (seven cerebrovascular events in controls vs. none in treated subjects; ten fatal and nonfatal coronary events in controls vs. 14 in treated subjects). The authors of the Oslo study stated that "Considering the mild degree of hypertension, the small size of the study groups and the short follow-up time, it was not unexpected that both total mortality and mortality from cardiovascular events were uninfluenced by drug treatment . . . valid conclusions regarding the impact of antihypertensive treatment on mortality should not be drawn." It is notable that no patient suffered from a stroke, and only five other vascular complications occurred in the treated group, compared with seven cases of stroke and 14 other vascular complications in the control group.

The MRC trial, which involved more than 17,000 patients randomized to receive placebo, propranolol, or a diuretic and followed up over a 5- to 6-year period, noted that approximately 15% to 20% of patients with less severe hypertension became and remained normotensive without specific therapy, usually within 3 months. Since these patients had been carefully screened before the study, it is probable that even a greater number of unselected mildly hypertensive patients will become normotensive without specific therapy—a strong argument for observation for a 3- to 4-month period before instituting therapy.

Although prerandomization blood pressure levels in the MRC trial group differed somewhat from those in the HDFP and Australian mild hypertensive subjects (90 to 109 mm Hg in MRC; 90 to 104 mm Hg in HDFP; 95 to 110 mm Hg in the Australian study), stroke event rates in the MRC treated patients were reduced to a degree equivalent to that in the other studies (45% reduction in both total and nontotal strokes in the treated MRC group; fatal strokes were reduced by 34%). In the MRC study, patients in the diuretic group experienced a greater fall in blood pressure and a greater decrease in strokes compared with the β-blocker–treated groups.

A statistically significant decrease in coronary events was not noted (especially in smokers), but the incidence of all cardiovascular events was decreased by 19% in the MRC treated group. This result is similar to that noted in the HDFP study, despite the differences in study design and population demographics.

Observations Regarding Therapy

In patients with mild hypertension who are generally asymptomatic and whose risk for an immediate cardiovascular incident is minimal, it is important that if pharmacologic therapy is to be used, we employ medications that will produce the fewest side effects and the fewest metabolic changes.

The Multiple Risk Factor Intervention Trial (MRFIT) provides an example of how physicians have responded to a study that was not specifically designed to assess the effectiveness of antihypertensive drug therapy. This was a 6- to 7-year trial involving a group of middle-aged men at high risk for cardiovascular disease. Its results have, in my opinion, been misinterpreted and used as an argument against treating patients with mild hypertension.

The unexpected findings in MRFIT were that cholesterol levels, smoking, and blood pressure levels were lowered not only in the group of men assigned to special intervention clinics (SI group) but also in the men referred back to their own physicians for usual care (UC group). It had been estimated, based on a risk factor profile, that a total of 442 deaths would occur in the UC group (187 of these from coronary disease) if, as anticipated, no reduction in blood pressure or lipid levels would occur. This was not the case. Only 260 men died; only 124 from coronary artery disease. The SI group had similar mortality findings, with a total of 265 deaths with only 115 from coronary artery disease. The differences between the groups were not statistically significant probably because the UC men had also had their blood pressures and cholesterol levels lowered to almost as great a degree as the SI men. The results of the MRFIT study actually confirmed that reduction of risk factors, whether in a physician's office or at special centers, reduces mortality.

In an attempt to explain the failure to demonstrate a significant difference in death rates between the two groups, subgroup analyses were done. These analyses revealed a subgroup of SI hypertensive patients with pretreatment abnormal ECGs in whom the death rate was higher than in a similar UC cohort. The investigators suggested that, despite the weakness of this type of analysis, some intervention had resulted in an increased mortality. There has been speculation that the use of diuretics could have contributed to this finding. We have analyzed the results of this study elsewhere and find little evidence to substantiate this interpretation.

Several unexplainable findings in the MRFIT study are of interest. (1) Patients in the UC group with abnormal pretreatment ECGs had an unusually low mortality (Table 6). All other studies have shown that hypertensive patients with abnormal pretreatment ECGs have a higher mortality than those with normal ECGs regardless of the type of management, yet the UC group did not show this. Could the increase in the SI group, then,

TABLE 6.
MRFIT: Subgroup Analyses for Deaths From Coronary Heart Disease

Subgroup	No. in Group		Rate, No. (%)	
	SI	UC	SI	UC
Hypertensive				
Resting ECG abnormalities	1,233	1,185	36 (29.2)	21 (17.7)
No resting ECG abnormalities	2,785	2,808	44 (15.8)	58 (20.7)

have been only a relative increase? (2) Patients receiving chlorthalidone had a lower mortality than those receiving hydrochlorothiazide, and yet both in the MRFIT and the previous studies, chlorthalidone caused a greater degree of hypokalemia than did hydrochlorothiazide. If hypokalemia is allegedly a factor in the increased mortality, this finding is difficult to explain. (3) Finally, in the group of men with abnormal pretreatment exercise stress test results, a group within which patients with ischemic heart disease should be found, deaths were lower, not higher, in the SI group. If therapy in the SI group had adversely affected outcome by causing hypokalemia and ventricular arrhythmias, as has been suggested, deaths in this subset of patients should have been higher than in the UC group.

Careful analyses have also failed to prove that there was a relationship between deaths and the dosage of diuretics. These data suggest, therefore, that speculations arising from the MRFIT results are not justified by the facts, and that suggested differences may have been caused by a statistical aberration.

The entire issue of risk-benefit of treating mildly hypertensive patients is further confused by the hypokalemia-ectopy debate. Several studies, apart from the MRFIT study, suggest an increased incidence of ventricular ectopy in patients with diuretic-induced hypokalemia. Others have failed to confirm these observations in hypertensive patients with or without evidence of left ventricular hypertrophy. Although a group of thiazide-treated patients from the MRC study demonstrated increased ectopy when compared with those receiving placebo, these patients were studied only after therapy; no baseline monitoring was undertaken. Before- and after-treatment monitoring in another group of patients did not confirm this finding. I do not believe that metabolic changes that may occur following the use of some of the drugs commonly used in treating mild hypertension (diuretics or β-blockers, for example) should deter physicians from treating mild hypertension with these agents.

The beneficial effects noted in the clinical trials are, in my opinion, enough to justify the treatment of the patient with mild hypertension, provided the treatment is kept simple and relatively inexpensive and the patient remains relatively free of side effects. I believe that this can be accomplished by the use of medications, as recently advocated by the Joint National Committee, specifically the use of diuretics as first-step therapy in the majority of patients and β-adrenergic inhibitors as first-step therapy in other specific patient groups.

In my experience, subjective side effects following the use of diuretics are relatively infrequent; rarely must another medication be substituted. Hypokalemia may be a problem in the elderly patient but is relatively uncommon in other patients. Titration of diuretics is easy, cost is relatively low, and patients, after blood pressure is controlled, may only have to be seen two or three times a year. In my judgment, this does not require a major commitment or expense on the patient's part—I do not believe that most patients with mild hypertension who are treated with low-dose diuretics and/or low-dose β-blockers or, in a few cases, converting enzyme inhibitors (CEIs) experience a significant decrease in the "quality of life." When other drugs are used as first-step therapy, however, treatment may become more expensive, titration to an appropriate dosage is often more difficult, and, especially with centrally acting drugs such as clonidine, guanabenz, or methyldopa, subjective side effects are more difficult to manage.

I do not agree with physicians who state that the treatment of hypertension is complicated, patient adherence is poor, and quality of life is dramatically changed in many instances. In treatment programs over the past 30 years, we have achieved a high rate of success (>80% of patients remain normotensive) with a low dropout rate by following the above simple program.

In deciding whether and how to treat patients with mild hypertension, we are left with the argument that millions of individuals would have to be treated to benefit a few. However, if we use the data from HDFP, which demonstrated a 20% decrease in mortality, over 46,000 lives can be saved each year by treating mild hypertension, and this is probably an underestimation of benefit (Table 7). This compares with a recent estimate of 10,000 lives saved each year in coronary care units in the United States. Data from the MRC and EWPHE trials are also of interest in calculating the potential benefit of therapy in both the patient with mild hypertension and the elderly hypertensive patient. A reduction of 1.2 stroke events or 1.6 cardiovascular events per 1,000 patient-years in the treated patients in the MRC study suggests a minimal benefit but in fact represents an overall reduction of 24,000 strokes or 32,000 cardiovascular events per year in the population of approximately 20 million mildly hypertensive patients in the United States. In the Australian trial there was a decrease in total fatal end points of only two per 1,000 patient-years in the treated patients—a potential decrease in deaths of 40,000 per year in the 20 million mildly

TABLE 7.
Estimates of Possible Benefits per Year From Treating Mild Hypertension

Study	Reduction Following Therapy	Reduction Assuming 20 Million Mildly Hypertensive U.S. Patients
HDFP	20% (2.3/1,000 patient-yr)	46,000 lives/yr
MRC	1.2 strokes/1,000 patient-yr	24,000 strokes
	1.6 cardiovascular events/ 1,000 patient-yr	32,000 events/yr
Australian trial	2 fatal end points/1,000 patient-yr	40,000 fatal events/yr
	7.3 fatal and nonfatal events	146,000 fatal and nonfatal events
Over 4 yr	10 deaths/1,721 patients	116,000 deaths
	20 nonfatal events/1,721 patients	232,000 morbid events
Over 20 yr	1 death/25 persons	800,000 deaths
	1 morbid event/7 persons	2,850,000 morbid events

hypertensive patients in the United States. The 7.3/1,000 patient-years reduction noted in total fatal and nonfatal end points in actively treated patients suggests benefit to 146,000 patients per year in the U.S. mildly hypertensive population. If we follow the argument of some investigators that 1,721 patients would have to be treated for four years to prevent or postpone ten deaths and 20 nonfatal morbid events (based on the Australian study), this suggests that 116,000 deaths and 232,000 morbid events could be prevented in the United States by treatment of mild hypertension. Finally, if these benefits were constant in the 20 million U.S. mildly hypertensive patients, with no improvement in outcome (which probably would actually occur), after 20 years of treatment the minimum benefit would be one in 25 for postponement of death (800,000 people) and one in seven for any significant morbid event (2,850,000 people). These are impressive numbers. The potential reduction in mortality alone would appear to make treatment of this entity worthwhile, without consideration of the reduction in morbidity or the potential benefits of preventing progression to severe hypertension or the undetectable vascular changes that may occur in untreated hypertensive subjects.

Based on data presented herein and on my own experience, patients with mild hypertension who have persistently elevated blood pressures over 140/90 mm Hg will benefit from therapy with specific antihypertensive medications. In addition, it is apparent that patients whose blood pressures are restored to normotensive levels will experience fewer cardiovascular complications than those whose blood pressures are not lowered to a goal of under 140/90 mm Hg.

Conclusions

Sufficient data have been accumulated to justify lowering blood pressure in patients with less severe degrees of hypertension (DBPs of 90 to 104 mm Hg). Although the immediate or even short-term risk of cardiovascular complications is not great in these patients, long-term risk is significantly increased compared with normotensive individuals. At present, it seems imprudent to await objective evidence of target-organ involvement before beginning therapy.

In this relatively low-risk group, blood pressure should be measured several times over a 3- to 6-month period to establish the diagnosis. Nonpharmacologic methods of treatment should be attempted before specific antihypertensive drug therapy is undertaken, although subsets of patients at higher risk should be treated sooner.

If nonpharmacologic methods are successful in maintaining DBP at levels under 90 mm Hg, they should be continued; if not, the SC method of therapy, utilizing a diuretic and/or one of several adrenergic-inhibiting drugs as initial therapy, will prove effective in a majority of patients. Side effects and cost of therapy should not be great in these individuals. Arguments against instituting therapy at these levels of pressure are based on theoretical implications of long-term toxic drug reaction, which, after 25 years of experience, has not been demonstrated.

Maintaining goal blood pressure over the long term in patients with less severe hypertension can be expected to decrease the incidence of cerebrovascular disease and of deaths from this cause. Furthermore, it can be expected to prevent progression to more severe hypertension, prevent left ventricular hypertrophy, and produce an overall decrease in deaths from cardiovascular and coronary heart disease.

Bibliography

1. Amery A, Birkenhoger W, Brixko D, et al: Mortality and morbidity results from the European Working Party on High Blood Pressure in the Elderly Trial. *Lancet* 1985; 1:1349–1354.
2. Helgeland A: Treatment of mild hypertension: A 5 year controlled drug trial: The Oslo Study. *Am J Med* 1980; 69:725–732.
3. Hypertension Detection and Follow-up Program: The effect of treatment on mortality in "mild" hypertension. *N Engl J Med* 1982; 307:967–980.

4. Management Committee: The Australian therapeutic trial in mild hypertension. *Lancet* 1980; 1:1261–1267.
5. Medical Research Council Working Party: MRC trial of treatment of mild hypertension: Principal results. *Br Med J* 1985; 291:97–104.
6. McAlister NH: Should we treat "mild" hypertension? *JAMA* 1983; 249:379–382.
7. Moser M: A decade of progress in the management of hypertension. *Hypertension* 1983; 5:808–813.
8. Moser M: Clinical trials and their effect on medical therapy: The Multiple Risk Factor Intervention Trial. *Am Heart J* 1984; 107:616–618.
9. Moser M, Gilford R: Why less severe degrees of hypertension should be treated. *J Hypertens* 1985; 3:437–447.
10. Papademetriou V, Fletcher R, Khatri IM, et al: Diuretic-induced hypokalemia in uncomplicated systemic hypertension: Effect of plasma potassium correction on cardiac arrhythmias. *Am J Cardiol* 1983; 52:1017–1022.
11. Stamler J: Epidemiology of hypertension: Achievements and challenges, in Moser M (ed): *Hypertension: A Practical Approach*. Boston, Little, Brown & Co, 1975.

Negative
Norman M. Kaplan, M.D.

As more of the 40 million people in the United States who have mild hypertension are identified, both they and their doctors seek an effective and easy way to reduce the elevated blood pressure. This way is increasingly through antihypertensive drugs, so that the treatment of hypertension is now the major indication for the use of prescription drugs in the United States. The use of such drugs will almost certainly continue to expand since easier to use and take medications are being constantly provided and aggressively marketed.

Although the appropriate application of antihypertensive drug therapy will unquestionably save lives by preventing the progress of cardiovascular diseases, I believe the use of these drugs is often unnecessary and occasionally harmful. They may be unnecessary for three reasons.

The Tendency for Pressures to Fall

First, many people's blood pressure will fall to levels that do not require treatment if repeated measurements are taken over 3 to 6 months after the recognition of their hypertension. Although there are some patients whose blood pressure is so high or whose risk for cardiovascular complications is so threatening that they require immediate treatment to lower their blood pressure, by far the majority of patients can safely be monitored for a few months without such treatment. Witness the experience of the non–drug-treated half of the patients enrolled in the Australian trial: 48% of the entire group with DBPs between 95 and 109 mm Hg on the second of two monthly sets of readings had readings persistently below 95 mm Hg for the next 4 years. Most of the fall in blood pressure, which averaged some 6.6 mm Hg for the entire population of non–drug-treated patients, occurred within the first 4 months after entry. Even among those with the highest range of initial DBP, from 105 to 109 mm Hg, the DBP of 11% remained below 90 mm Hg while receiving *no drugs* for the remainder of the trial. Admittedly, 12% of the entire placebo-treated half had a rise in DBP to above 100 mm Hg during the trial so that they had to be started on drug therapy.

The point should be clear: all found to be hypertensive should be kept under surveillance but many will be found who do not need active drug therapy. The most efficient way to monitor most people is by multiple measurements taken at home by the patient with semiautomatic blood pressure devices readily available for around $65. In the future, one set of ambulatory 24-hour readings taken with an automatic device may prove to be adequate screening, compressed into a much shorter time. Regardless of how they are obtained, many readings taken under diverse circumstances will provide better evidence of the true and persistent nature of the blood pressure than will multiple readings taken only in the doctor's office. But even if only office readings are practical, many of them—at the least three sets on three separate occasions, preferably 1 month apart—should be obtained, to document the natural tendency for the pressure to fall in many people or to ensure that the patient's range of pressure is high enough to mandate drug therapy.

The Degree of Risk

The second reason drug therapy may be unnecessary is that many people found to stay hypertensive most of the time will not have readings high enough to mandate drug therapy. The blood pressure level that is associated with an increased *relative risk* is actually quite low for the population at large. However, when considering the *absolute risk* for an individual patient, that level of pressure may pose only a small danger. Thus, among the 7,054 men, 40 to 59 years old, who were followed up for an average of 8.6 years in the Pooling Project, the relative risk for developing coronary disease increased by 52% for those with initial DBP from 80 to 87 mm Hg compared with that for those with DBP below 80 mm Hg (Table 8). However, that 52% increase in relative risk actually translates to an increase in

---

TABLE 8.
Risk for Major Coronary Events in 7,054 White Men by DBP at Entry*

DBP at Entry†	Adjusted Rate of Major Coronary Events per 1,000	Relative Risk	Absolute Excess Risk per 1,000
Below 80 (quintiles 1 and 2)	66.0	1.0	. . .
80–87 (quintile 4)	100.6	1.52	34.6
88–95 (quintile 4)	109.4	1.66	43.4
Above 95 (quintile 5)	143.3	2.17	77.3

*From the Pooling Project Research Group: Relationship of blood pressure, serum cholesterol, and smoking habit. *J Chronic Dis* 1978; 31:201. Reproduced by permission. Risk over 8.6 years.
†The blood pressure ranges varied slightly for various 5-year age groups: 40 to 44, 45 to 49, etc.

absolute risk for developing coronary disease from seven up to ten men per 100 over the next 8.6 years.

Many have taken the level of 90 mm Hg for DBP as being associated with enough risk to mandate institution of drug therapy. Others, mainly outside the United States, have insisted on readings of 100 mm Hg or higher. I believe the level of 95 mm Hg, as the average reading after at least 3 months of repeated measurements, is a reasonable compromise. This is the conclusion reached by an expert committee of the World Health Organization and International Society of Hypertension (WHO/ISH).

Another element should enter into the decision: the patient's overall cardiovascular risk status. Those at high risk, such as diabetics with microalbuminuria, should probably be treated if they have DBP above 85 mm Hg or even lower levels. Those at low risk, for example, older women with none of the other known risk factors, such as hypercholesterolemia, smoking, and diabetes, may safely be left off drug therapy even with somewhat higher readings.

The preceding has considered only DBPs. The same arguments can be applied to systolic readings, with the important proviso that most who have isolated systolic hypertension are elderly, and we have no good evidence about the safety or effectiveness of treating them at present. Until the results of the Systolic Hypertension in the Elderly Program become available, I believe a gentle, gradual reduction in systolic blood pressure to below 160 mm Hg is probably worthwhile in most people at any age.

The Value of Nondrug Therapies

The third reason that drug treatment may be unnecessary is that nondrug therapies may bring the pressure down to a safe level. These should be tried by all patients, even if they also need drugs, but particularly by the majority of hypertensive people who have such minimally elevated pressure that even a little nudge downward will be enough.

A number of points about nondrug therapies need to be recognized. They have not been, and likely never will be, shown to reduce the risks for cardiovascular disease. They are less potent than antihypertensive drugs, and, as we shall recall, it has not been possible to show protection against coronary disease among mildly hypertensive patients with drugs. To expect better with nondrug therapy—more difficult to monitor and less potent—is both unnecessary and irrational.

Even if ineffectual in lowering blood pressure, nondrug therapies should improve the patient's overall cardiovascular risk status. Proper diet, exercise, and moderation of alcohol use are good for everyone, hypertensive or not.

Their use should be comfortable, convenient, and with no conceivable risk. Applied with good sense and concern for patients' life style, they should not be a burden.

If advocated with enthusiasm, prescribed in a reasonable manner, and monitored by appropriate means, nondrug therapies will likely be used by about as many people as will drug therapy. But care should be taken not to oversell or overdo these therapies. Sodium restriction need only be to a level of 80 to 100 mmol/day, half the usual American intake. Exercise need only be for 30 minutes three times a week, as long as it is isotonic and fairly vigorous. However, the exercise should be enjoyable or at least easily tolerated or it may be deleted from the nondrug prescription (Table 9). Most of the items given in Table 9 have been shown in properly controlled trials to lower the blood pressure by 5 to 10 mm Hg in many patients, at least for 6 months. Longer trials are under way.

The Risks of Drug Therapy

Beyond the fact that drugs may be unnecessary, too fast and too broad use of antihypertensive drugs may expose millions of people to both discomfort and additional risks. I will review first the evidence that drug therapy, as has commonly been used, has likely increased the risks for coronary disease, at least among an important segment of the hypertensive population. Then I will examine the evidence that, whatever their effects on cardiovascular risk, all of the drugs used to treat hypertension may cause adverse effects and interfere with the quality of life.

Results of Clinical Trials

Six large clinical trials have examined the question: will antihypertensive drug therapy of patients with mild hypertension protect them against major

---

TABLE 9.
Nondrug Therapy for Hypertension

If obese, weight reduction
Dietary sodium restricted to 2 gm/day (88 mmol/day)
More fiber and less saturated fat
Supplemental potassium, magnesium, and calcium if deficiency exists
Alcohol limited to 2 oz/day
Regular isotonic exercise
Relaxation therapy

---

cardiovascular complications? Four of these were straightforward placebo vs. drug trials (Table 10). The results of these trials showed clear protection against death from stroke as well as against progression of the level of blood pressure. But for coronary mortality—by far the major cardiovascular complication faced by all people in industrialized societies, whether hypertensive or not—protection has not been uniformly found. When the results of these individual trials are added up, the incidence of coronary mortality is found not to be significantly reduced.

The other two trials, both done in the United States, offered therapy to all of the subjects but allocated the patients to receive the therapy either in a more intensive or "special" manner vs. a less intensive or "usual" manner. In these two trials, protection against coronary mortality was found for those patients who entered with normal ECGs (Table 11). However, among the more than one third of the subjects whose entry ECG was in any way abnormal, higher rates of subsequent coronary mortality were found among those who were more intensively treated.

Two special aspects of these trials should be kept in mind. First, diuretics, often in high doses, were the first drug used in all of the trials with one partial exception: in the MRC trial, a β-blocker was given to half of the drug-treated group. No only were diuretics the first drug used, they were often the only drug needed. Since the trials involved patients with mild hypertension, the first drug was adequate to bring the blood pressure down to the goal of therapy in about half of all subjects. Almost all who needed more drugs continued on the diuretic therapy as well. Moreover, the doses of diuretic were often, by today's standards, rather high: up to 100 mg/day of chlorthalidone or hydrochlorothiazide.

Second, these studies were begun in the early 1970s, at a time when most of the biochemical side effects of diuretics were either unrecognized,

---

TABLE 10.
Results of Four Placebo-Controlled Trials of the Drug Treatment of Mild Hypertension

| | Mortality per 1,000 Person-yr | | | | | |
| | Cerebrovascular Disease | | | Coronary Heart Disease | | |
Trial, yr	Placebo	Drug	Difference, %	Placebo	Drug	Difference, %
Australia, 1980	0.9	0.4	−56	1.6	0.7	−56
Oslo, 1980	1.0	0	−100	1.0	2.7	+170
MRC, 1985	0.6	0.4	−33	2.3	2.5	+9
EWPHE, 1985	16	11	−32	24	15	−38

TABLE 11.
Results of Two Trials of the Drug Treatment of Mild
Hypertension

| Trial | No. of Subjects | Coronary Heart Disease Rate per 1,000 Person-yr | | |
		Less Therapy	More Therapy	Difference, %
HDFP				
Normal ECG	3,210	3.1	2.0	−35
Abnormal ECG	1,963	3.5	4.3	+23
MRFIT				
Normal ECG	5,593	3.4	2.6	−24
Abnormal ECG	2,418	2.9	4.9	+70

e.g., hypercholesterolemia, or considered to be harmless, e.g., hypokalemia. As would be expected with fairly large doses of diuretic, hypokalemia was frequent, and hypercholesterolemia, when looked for, often occurred at least initially.

I believe these and other diuretic-induced biochemical side effects, such as glucose intolerance and hypomagnesemia, may very well have been responsible for the lack of protection against coronary disease observed. Most of the coronary mortality in the treated half were sudden deaths, caused by ventricular arrhythmias. Today, diuretic-induced hypokalemia has been clearly though not universally recognized to be responsible for increased ventricular ectopic activity. The potential for serious arrhythmias is particularly heightened in those with abnormal heart size, conduction, or rhythm preceding therapy. Witness the HDFP and MRFIT trials (see Table 11), wherein the excess coronary mortality was seen among those who received more intensive, i.e., diuretic, therapy only if they entered the trials with an abnormal ECG.

These two points are iterated because they likely explain why drug therapy *as used in these trials* did not protect against, and may have even worsened, the risk for coronary disease. Would other drugs do better? Unfortunately, there is little evidence to provide an answer. The half of the patients who were given a β-blocker (propranolol) in the MRC trial did no better overall, with the exception of the men who did not smoke cigarettes, who did have less coronary disease compared with those given a diuretic. A similar selective protection against coronary disease by another β-blocker, oxprenolol, was observed only in men who did not smoke cigarettes in another trial, the International Prospective Primary Prevention Study in Hypertension (IPPPSH) study, designed specifically to examine the value of the β-blocker.

With these two exceptions, wherein β-blockers appear to protect in one portion of the hypertensive population, there is no other evidence that other forms of antihypertensive therapy will do any better than will diuretics. Knowing that other drugs will not cause hypokalemia, hypercholesterolemia, and glucose intolerance, I think it reasonable that they would provide more protection against coronary disease. However, we will probably never know. Trials adequate to provide the answer will likely never be done with α-blockers, CEIs, and calcium entry blockers, the other three main classes of antihypertensive drugs now available. Nonetheless, their use as initial therapy in more and more patients with mild hypertension can be defended on the basis of their lesser propensity to cause potentially harmful biochemical changes while providing equal antihypertensive efficacy.

Adverse Effects

This advocacy of other drugs should be tempered by the realization that they too may cause adverse effects. There is no antihypertensive drug that causes no side effects and there probably never will be one. Some of these side effects reflect the intrinsic manner of action of the drugs to lower the blood pressure. Flushing and fluid retention as seen with vasodilators, sedation and dry mouth as seen with central α-agonists, fatigue and depression as seen with β-blockers may be part of the necessary baggage carried by these agents as they lower the blood pressure.

In the previously described clinical trials, 20% to 40% of patients experienced drug side effects, very rarely serious but bothersome nonetheless. And these trials were carefully designed and monitored. The likelihood for mischief from drugs is even greater in ordinary clinical practice. To be sure, the adverse effects of antihypertensive therapy can be reduced by more careful use of what is available and by choosing those drugs less likely to cause side effects. For example, carefully performed trials have documented less interference with the quality of life by CEIs than with β-blockers and central α-agonists (methyldopa). But as benign as CEIs may be, they too may cause adverse effects. Simply put, there is today no free lunch when using antihypertensive drug therapy.

Conclusion

Drug therapy for hypertension may be lifesaving. However, not all people with mild hypertension need to be given drugs to lower their blood pressure. Even if nondrug therapies don't work completely, they will probably reduce overall cardiovascular risk and may preclude the need for drugs. Many with minimally elevated pressure are not at enough risk to mandate therapy that carries some risk along with its potential benefits.

Better and safer drugs are now available, so the balance between risk and benefit will likely tip increasingly toward benefit. Regardless, in our therapeutic enthusiasm to do something, we must avoid doing harm while we are trying to do good.

Bibliography

1. Amery A, Birkenhager W, Brixko P, et al: Mortality and morbidity results from the European Working Party on High Blood Pressure in the Elderly Trial. *Lancet* 1985; 1:1349–1354.
2. Croog SH, Levine S, Testa MA, et al: The effects of antihypertensive therapy on the quality of life. *N Engl J Med* 1986; 314:1657–1664.
3. Helgeland A: Treatment of mild hypertension: A 5 year controlled drug trial: The Oslo Study. *Am J Med* 1980; 69:725–732.
4. Helgeland A, Strømmen R, Hagelund CH, et al: Enalapril, atenolol, and hydrochlorothiazide in mild to moderate hypertension. *Lancet* 1986; 1:872–875.
5. Kaplan NM: Non-drug treatment of hypertension. *Ann Intern Med* 1985; 102:359–373.
6. Kaplan NM: Treatment of hypertension: Nondrug therapy and the rationale for drug therapy, in Kaplan NM (ed): *Clinical Hypertension*, ed 4. Baltimore, Williams & Wilkins Co, 1986, pp 147–179.
7. Kuller LH, Hulley SB, Cohen JD, et al: Unexpected effects of treating hypertension in men with electrocardiographic abnormalities: A critical analysis. *Circulation* 1986; 73:114–123.
8. Management Committee: The Australian therapeutic trial in mild hypertension. *Lancet* 1980; 1:1261–1267.
9. Medical Research Council Working Party: MRC trial of treatment of mild hypertension: Principal results. *Br Med J* 1985; 291:97–104.
10. Subcommittee on Nonpharmacological Therapy of the 1984 Joint National Committee on Detection, Evaluation and Treatment of High Blood Pressure: Nonpharmacological approaches to the control of high blood pressure. *Hypertension* 1986; 8:444–467.
11. The IPPPSH Collaborative Group: Cardiovascular risk and risk factors in a randomized trial of treatment based on the β-blocker oxprenolol: The International Prospective Primary Prevention Study in Hypertension (IPPPSH). *J Hypertens* 1985; 3:379–392.
12. The Pooling Project Research Group: Relationship of blood pressure, serum cholesterol, smoking habit, relative weight and ECG abnormalities to incidence of major coronary events: Final report of the Pooling Project. *J Chronic Dis* 1978; 31:201–306.
13. WHO/ISH: 1986 guidelines for the treatment of mild hypertension: Memorandum from a WHO/ISH meeting. *J Hypertens* 1986; 4:383–386.

Rebuttal: Affirmative

Marvin Moser, M.D.

It is important to put into perspective Dr. Kaplan's arguments against the widespread use of drug therapy in the treatment of mild hypertension.

I believe that the estimate of 40 million mildly hypertensive patients in the United States is based on studies that, on review, I do not consider accurate. It is more probable that the actual number of mildly hypertensive patients is closer to 20 to 25 million. If so, this lower estimate reduces the number of potential candidates for drug therapy.

I would agree with Dr. Kaplan, and have so stated, that mildly hypertensive patients should be followed up for at least 3 to 6 months before the institution of specific antihypertensive drug therapy. The risk for cardiovascular complications is not great in these patients, and this period of observation allows for a trial of nonpharmacologic therapy. However, it is my belief that a far lower percentage than the 48% quoted by Dr. Kaplan (based on the Australian trial) will revert to normotensive levels. Abernathy,[1] in discussing this statement, advised that this number may not be correct and "was based upon a retrospective analysis of a selected sample." For example, Dr. Kaplan's estimate included approximately 237 borderline subjects (a special subgroup whose pressures fell after meeting the admissions criteria and who were randomized but eliminated from the final analysis after consistently remaining below the prescribed 95 mm Hg for being given placebo tablets). Excluded from the denominator of this number were all those with cardiovascular end points and those whose pressures rose to DBPs above 115 mm Hg, plus those subjects who did not comply at 3 years. This included as many as 33% of the 1,943 randomized placebo-treated patients. Although the progressive fall to more normal pressure levels has been demonstrated in most clinical trials, I doubt that the percentage of patients is anywhere near the 48% suggested by Dr. Kaplan.

I take exception to the statement that ambulatory blood pressure monitoring for 24 hours might provide adequate screening for the group who might not require therapy. Nor would I accept the data from these recordings as an index of risk; all information regarding the risk of hypertension for cardiovascular disease and, in fact, data from the clinical trials on which we base our decisions to treat depend on a series of casual blood pressures in a doctor's office or clinic. There is no information to suggest that 24-hour monitoring is of prognostic value. The data quoted from the Pooling Project do appear to overstate the absolute risk to an individual for developing coronary artery disease when pressures of below 80 mm Hg are compared with DBPs of 80 to 87 mm Hg. However, these data also established that the absolute risk of developing coronary disease increased from seven to more than 14 per 100 when diastolic pressures were above 95 mm Hg and from seven to 11 per 100 when diastolic pressures of 88 to 95 mm Hg were compared with those below 80 mm Hg. If we extrapolate these numbers (at the 88 to 95 mm Hg level) to only a possible 10 million mildly hypertensive persons in the United States, the risk becomes considerable and includes 434,000 men over an 8.6-year period. If we use Dr. Kaplan's estimate of 40 million mildly hypertensive persons, the number is 1,736,000. This represents a considerable public health as well as an individual risk.

There is no question that other cardiovascular risk factors should enter into the decision as to when and how to treat mild hypertension. An obese 57-year-old diabetic man with mild hypertension (140/90 to 155/100 mm Hg) should be treated more readily than a 41-year-old thin, white woman with no other cardiovascular risks. As we noted in our original discussion, in our experience, treatment with nonpharmacologic measures has not been successful in a significant number of patients. I would argue that there is also an inconvenience and a risk to nonpharmacologic intervention and concur with Dr. Freis'[2] recent review that at present the data on sodium restriction, for example, do not indicate that this should be a definitive treatment of hypertension. Indeed, a recent review from the National High Blood Pressure Coordinating Council on Nonpharmacologic Therapies in Hypertension reaches a similar conclusion.[3]

I disagree, as pointed out in my position paper, with some of Dr. Kaplan's interpretation of the clinical trials. I find it difficult to understand why statistical significance was omitted from Table 10: which suggests that treatment did not decrease mortality from coronary heart disease. A suggestion that the risk of coronary disease in treated patients is increased by 170% (as Dr. Kaplan suggests was found in the Oslo study), if statistically valid, would be an important observation. However, I must point out that the authors of the Oslo study themselves noted (at 5 years) that the numbers were small (6 vs. 2) and failed to achieve statistical significance, and they warned that conclusions based on their data should not be drawn. If Dr. Kaplan wishes to use the 10-year Oslo data[4] (14 deaths in treated vs. three in control subjects), I also must point out that these are death registry data only and that *no information on treatment or morbidity* were available in these patients from the fifth to the tenth year. It is quite possible that more than half the control subjects were treated by their physicians or that more than half of the treated patients were withdrawn from therapy, etc. In the MRC trial, the difference between placebo and treated groups in regard to coronary heart disease was also not statistically significant. It is important that clinical trial results be put in perspective and judged based on statistical significance, not on findings that might happen by chance.

Omitted from Table 10 is the HDFP study, which, although not including a placebo or control group (the Oslo study did not have a placebo group but had a control or no-treatment group), is a valid study that clearly demonstrated the benefits of a greater decrease in blood pressure in a higher percentage of people in the vigorously treated group. Deaths from cerebrovascular *and* cardiovascular and coronary disease were reduced. We should also emphasize the positive results of the EWPHE study, which were significant.

Speculations that revolve around the possible deleterious effects of the medications used in clinical trials are merely that.

I have reviewed the MRFIT study in detail in my original discussion. I have great difficulty in reconciling the argument that diuretics (in low or high doses) may increase mortality in some patients because of adverse metabolic effects (on potassium or lipids) with the fact that the chlorthalidone-treated patients had a significantly *lower* mortality than the hydrochlorothiazide-treated patients.[5] Yet hypokalemia was present to a greater degree with chlorthalidone, and there is no reason to believe that lipid changes were less with this drug when compared with hydrochlorothiazide. The MRFIT study indicates that high-dose chlorthalidone users (with more hypokalemia?) had the lowest death rate (Table 12).

With regard to the HDFP study, the authors of this study, in comparing mortality findings in an HDFP subgroup (similar to MRFIT patients), with and without ECG abnormalities, report a reduction in all causes of mortality in those patients with ECG abnormalities. Unlike the MRFIT cohort, patients with resting ECG abnormalities before treatment had a higher, not a lower, mortality, whether they were in the less vigorously or the more vigorously treated group. This is consistent with studies other than MRFIT and, as noted, may explain the aberrance of the MRFIT data. The HDFP

TABLE 12.
MRFIT: Mortality and Diuretic Dose*

Diuretic Dose, mg/ day	SI Group Mortality	
	Abnormal ECG	Normal ECG
Chlorthalidone	3.31	2.08
<50	4.84	1.76
>50	1.84	2.37
HCTZ	7.61	2.21
<50	7.20	2.27
>50	8.01	2.55

*From MRFIT Study.
SI indicates special intervention; HCTZ indicates hydrochlorothiazide. Mortality is per 1,000 patient-years.

authors are careful to point out that the findings reported from MRFIT are particularly subject

to the play of random variation in the subgroups under consideration given the small number of deaths. . . . In MRFIT there is also the unexpected finding of a lower coronary heart disease mortality rate in hypertensive men receiving usual care, for those with resting ECG abnormalities than those free from it. This too could be caused by chance, given the small number of events. So that the apparent excess mortality from MRFIT hypertensive men in the special intervention group with ECG abnormalities may be artifactual.[6]

The differences noted in Dr. Kaplan's Table 11 are not of statistical significance.

I would agree with Dr. Kaplan's comments regarding the MRC trial, the IPPPSH trial, and the recently reported HAPPY study,[7] which showed little or no difference in overall cardiovascular mortality when diuretic-treated patients were compared with β-blocker–treated patients. Although the designs of these studies are different, the results are important.

One final comment: in our experience, fewer than 20% of patients receiving drug therapy experience significant or annoying side effects. This is probably because we have used few centrally acting adrenergic inhibitors, α-blockers, etc., as first-step therapy. Dr. Kaplan is, of course, correct: it is possible that utilization of other medications as first-step therapy *may* result in a further decrease in mortality and morbidity in the future, but at present we have no data to substantiate this. The arguments advanced by him have not, however, changed my approach to patients with persistently elevated blood pressure (>140/90 mm Hg) after a suitable period and after a trial of non-pharmacologic therapy. These patients should be treated with medication. If this is done carefully, the benefit both to the individual and to the population at large will be considerable.

References

1. Abernathy JD: The Australlian Therapeutic Trial in Mild Hypertension. *Hypertension* 1984; 6:774–776.
2. Freis E: Does moderate sodium restriction lower blood pressure? *Hypertension* 1986; 8:265–266.
3. *Non-pharmacologic Approaches to the Control of High Blood Pressure,* U.S. Dept of Health and Human Services publication, 1986.
4. Leren P, Helgeland, A: Oslo Hypertension Study. *Drugs* 1986; 31(suppl 1):41–45.
5. Bartsch GE, Broste S, Grandits GA, et al: Hydrochlorothiazide, chlorthalidone and mortality in the Multiple Risk Factor Intervention Trial. *Circulation* 1984; 70(suppl 2):360.
6. The Hypertension Detection and Follow-up Program Cooperative Research Group: The effect of antihypertensive drug treatment on mortality in the pres-

ence of resting electrocardiographic abnormalities at baseline: The HDFP experience. *Circulation* 1984; 70:996–1003.

7. Wilhelmsen L, Berglund G, Elmfeldt D, et al: Beta blockers vs diuretics in hypertension. Results of the Heart Attack Primary Prevention in Hypertension Trial Group (HAPPY). *Hypertension* 1987; 5:561–574.

Rebuttal: Negative
Norman M. Kaplan, M.D.

Dr. Moser and I have some fundamentally different opinions, perhaps best expressed around his statement: "Data indicate that the benefit of treatment outweighs the risk and that blood pressure can be lowered with relatively few adverse reactions or metabolic changes in most patients and with little effect on life-style."

I disagree with all three points. First, the benefit of treatment has not been shown to outweight risk in the large number of people—perhaps 40% of the hypertensive population—with DBPs between 90 and 95 mm Hg. As noted in Tables 10 and 11 of my article, *higher* death rates from coronary disease were reported in two of the four placebo-controlled studies and the one third or more of patients in both the HDFP and MRFIT studies who started the trials with an abnormal ECG and who received more intensive therapy. Once again, this does not discount the other benefits of therapy, specifically the reduction in stroke mortality. However, we need to be aware of the potential risks of our past therapies, as well as their potential benefits.

Second, although I agree that blood pressure can be lowered with relatively few adverse reactions or metabolic changes in many patients, the most carefully designed studies, such as that of Croog et al. in 1986, show that a large portion of patients will have adverse reactions with one of the three main classes of drugs now available (Table 13).

TABLE 13.
Effects of Three Antihypertensive Drugs on Quality of Life*

	Captopril	Methyldopa	Propranolol
No. of patients treated	213	201	212
No. of adverse reactions	30	89	51
No. of withdrawals due to adverse reactions	17	39	27
Percent requiring diuretic to control blood pressure	33	28	22

*From Croog: *N Engl J Med* 1986; 314:1657. Reproduced by permission.

Third, the effect of medications on life-style or "the quality of life" needs to be carefully considered. Whereas Croog et al. found that 51.4% of those given the angiotensin-converting enzyme (ACE) inhibitor reported an improved sense of general well-being, another 30.9% felt worse. Fewer felt better and more felt worse with propranolol and even more so with methyldopa. The addition of a diuretic to control the blood pressure, as noted in Table 13 to be needed in 22% to 33% of the patients, markedly reduced the overall feelings of well-being with all three of the drugs.

Let me briefly address a few other specific points made by Dr. Moser. He states that with the appropriate use of various nondrug therapies "it is conceivable that another 15% to 20% of patients will become normotensive." We really have no data on the "response rate" to multiple nondrug therapies, but many individually have been shown to lower blood pressures by at least 5 mm Hg for 1 to 6 months. Whether additional lowering is possible with multiple therapies and whether it will persist over longer times remains uncertain.

Dr. Moser cites the progression of hypertension, noted in over 10% of the nontreated group in the major clinical trials, as an indication for early therapy. I certainly advocate careful surveillance of all people with even one isolated high reading, but it seems inappropriate to treat everyone "early," since at least an equally large number will have a fall in DBP to below 90 mm Hg that, as shown in the Australian trial, will stay down for at least the next 4 years.

Dr. Moser suggests that if therapy is given before vascular target-organ damage appears "complications are fewer" than if given after damage has occurred. We do not know if early therapy will necessarily protect all patients equally. In the IPPPSH trial and the European trial in the elderly, the rate of complications was not related to the initial level of blood pressure but rather to the level of blood pressure achieved during the trial. Those whose pressure is more resistant to therapy thus may not be able to be protected, and it is that subgroup that contributes the largest number of complications. Early therapy may then not necessarily offer greater protection for the majority of patients who do not have a more resistant form of hypertension and a greater propensity for target-organ damage.

We really have no way to be sure which patient with fairly mild hypertension will develop target-organ damage and which will not. Obviously more damage will occur in those with more risk factors such as high cholesterol and glucose intolerance, and they should be treated more quickly than those with fewer risk factors. However, remember that the two most common forms of antihypertensive therapy, diuretics and β-blockers without intrinsic sympathic activity (ISA), may both raise lipid levels and worsen glucose tolerance.

Without going further into more of Dr. Moser's arguments, I would reaffirm my agreement with the 1986 recommendations of the WHO/ISH expert committee: treat with drugs those whose diastolic pressure remains above 95 mm Hg after at least 3 months of repeated measurements and appropriate nondrug therapy. There is little to gain and more to lose by a more aggressive approach in misdiagnosed and mistreated patients.

Editor's Comments
Nicholas J. Fortuin, M.D.

These two papers describe well the divergent positions of two experts on when and why to intervene with medication in patients with mild hypertension. Both authors stress the need for adequate documentation of elevated blood pressure on several determinations before embarking on any treatment. Both also emphasize the importance of nonpharmacologic therapy. They agree that treatment of mild cases may prevent progression to more severe hypertension, but Dr. Kaplan believes that observation will identify those who will progress and treatment can be started when there are indications of progression. Dr. Moser supports his position on early treatment by reviewing many studies that show a decrease in cardiovascular mortality in those treated aggressively. For Dr. Kaplan the evidence is less persuasive, and he emphasizes the fact that has confounded many who study this problem, namely, that treatment of even more severe hypertension has not lowered mortality from the most common disease associated with elevated blood pressure—coronary artery disease—in most studies. In fact, it is distressing that there are implications that mortality from this disease may be increased in those treated. It is reasonable to ask whether longer-term studies would produce different results, but the evidence at hand does not support the view that mortality from coronary artery disease can be lowered by early treatment of hypertension.

Germane to the issue of early treatment is the question of what drugs do to the patient. Dr. Moser notes that in his experience most patients can be managed without unpleasant side effects. Here Dr. Kaplan also differs, finding drug therapy difficult for many patients. The long-term consequences on electrolytes, glucose metabolism, and lipid metabolism of what for many may be lifelong drug therapy are not yet known. Potential deleterious consequences in these areas make me a cautious initiator of drug therapy in line with Dr. Kaplan's position. Perhaps newer drugs will have fewer side effects, but this information is not yet available. The physician still must decide whether to use diuretics, β-blockers, calcium channel blockers, or angiotensin-converting enzyme inhibitors without good understanding of what the long-term risk is with any of those agents.

I suspect that the question posed by this debate will rage for many years until better data are available to describe the risk-benefit ratio for long-term drug treatment. It is to be hoped that future studies will describe subgroups of patients with mild hypertension who will benefit from treatment so that therapeutic efforts can be directed at appropriate patients and not just at blood pressure numbers.

Sclerotherapy Is the Treatment of Choice for Esophageal Varices

Chapter Editor: Thomas P. Duffy, M.D.

Affirmative: Rosemarie Fisher, M.D.
Associate Professor of Medicine,
Gastroenterology Unit, Yale University
School of Medicine,
New Haven, Connecticut

Negative: Richard J. Gusberg, M.D.
Associate Professor of Surgery, Department
of General and Vascular Surgery, Yale
University School of Medicine,
New Haven, Connecticut

Debates in Medicine 1:64–85, 1988
©1988, Year Book Medical Publishers, Inc.
0887-218X/88/01-064-85-$04.00

Affirmative
Rosemarie Fisher, M.D.

The cirrhotic patient with portal hypertension often presents some of the most difficult therapeutic problems to the practicing clinician: ascites, encephalopathy, metabolic derangements, renal failure, and variceal hemorrhage. A cirrhotic patient with hematemesis arriving in an emergency room immediately faces an overall mortality risk of 22% to 84%. We know that this is not all due to hemorrhage in itself, but that mortality is primarily related to the severity of the underlying hepatocellular disease. However, the dramatic appearance of the exsanguinating patient makes all else appear secondary. The immediate response is to stop the bleeding and then to prevent the recurrence of hemorrhage. In the progression, then, of the therapy for hemorrhage from varices, one must look at measures to stop the active bleeding and, separately, measures to prevent its recurrence.

In addition, there is a separate issue that should be addressed: the prophylactic treatment of esophageal varices to prevent the first variceal hemorrhage. The prediction of variceal hemorrhage in an individual patient is complicated and difficult, involving local factors in the esophagus, portal pressure, variceal pressure, variceal size, variceal wall tension, blood volume, and ascites. However, because of the high mortality from the initial variceal hemorrhage (up to 30%) and the high costs of hospitalization, it appears appropriate to consider an effective therapy to prevent the initial hemorrhage.

Methods to stop and prevent variceal hemorrhage have traversed every medical specialty (medical, surgical, radiologic), and the pendulum has swung back and forth in the use of these procedures from the early 1900s to the present. In fact, the complications of the procedures performed years ago have not differed tremendously from the reported complications of the first portacaval shunt in a human in 1903—complications that still occur in present-day surgery for portal hypertension. The problem inherent in any therapy for variceal hemorrhage is that it will stop the hemorrhage (or possibility of rebleeding) by either occluding the bleeding vessel or decreasing the pressure in the portal system, thus reducing the pressure in the varices and reducing the chance of hemorrhage, but the therapy does nothing to alter the course of the primary liver disease and may even accentuate some of the other systemic complications (e.g., encephalopathy). The only true, complete cure of the ravages of chronic liver disease and portal hypertension appears to be liver transplantation. However, since this is not a realistic solution for the vast number of patients with portal hypertension, we must deal with what is available to the clinician.

The clinician who is faced with the cirrhotic patient with esophageal varices, both those that have bled and those that have yet to rupture, has several options: surgical therapy, angiographic therapy, pharmacologic therapy, or endoscopic therapy. Balloon tamponade (either with a Sengstaken-Blakemore tube or a Linton tube) remains in the clinical armamentarium, but as its role is temporary and acute, it only needs to be said that this will effectively stop the hemorrhage in about 75% of patients, but with a 45% incidence of recurrent hemorrhage.

Surgery

Surgical decompression of portosystemic collaterals has become the gold standard for treating these bleeding vessels. In fact, the clinical introduction of the portacaval anastomosis in 1946 by Blakemore was probably the reason that injection sclerotherapy of esophageal varices (first reported by Crafoord and Frenckner in 1939) was abandoned. Over the years, the enthusiasm for the portacaval shunt has waned. We now know that emergency shunt surgery has an unacceptably high mortality in the hands of most surgeons. The best results have been obtained in San Diego by Orloff,[17] where patients proceed to the operating room within 8 hours of presentation. However, even in this situation there is 40% mortality—still unacceptable. After several studies showing high mortality with emergency shunts, the practice changed to the initial stabilization of the patient, followed by a therapeutic shunt—either total or selective (distal splenorenal). The elective total (portacaval) shunts, however, when compared with medical therapy, were never documented to afford any long-term benefit in survival. Although this may have been difficult to show because of the variety of the studies, types of liver disease, Child's classification of patients, time of entry into study after hemorrhage, etc., it was thought that there was an increased morbidity and mortality in the shunted group because of a total diversion of portal venous blood flow from the liver. The "side-to-side" portacaval shunt attempted to correct this by maintaining portal venous flow to the liver. However, survival has not been shown to be better than the standard "end-to-side" portacaval shunt and may in fact be worse.

Attempts to refine the surgical procedure resulted in the splenorenal shunts. With these shunts, it was attempted selectively to decompress the gastroesophageal varices while maintaining the nutritive portal venous inflow to the liver. In this way, it was hoped that the incidence of hepatic encephalopathy, one of the most devastating effects of shunting, would be decreased. The most recent shunt of this type proposed is the distal splenorenal shunt, known as the Warren shunt. With this shunt, the gastric and esophageal varices are decompressed, but the portal venous flow to the liver is maintained. However, encephalopathy still occurs (reported as 12% in the initial studies), the incidence being no different from that with the total shunt in a recently completed randomized trial from New Haven,

Connecticut, and Boston. These data seem to disprove the theoretical advantages of the selective shunt. In addition, the distal splenorenal shunt is technically difficult and not performed adequately by all surgeons. Thus, though the shunt has remained the gold standard for the long-term treatment of variceal hemorrhage, the complications, mortality, and technical difficulty of the procedures have made physicians search for other possibilities.

Nondecompressive surgical methods have also been utilized. Ligation of esophageal varices had been performed since about 1953, as a temporizing measure, to stop variceal hemorrhage acutely and allow for stabilizing the patient. However, this needed to be performed through a thoracotomy, and there was high mortality and morbidity. In 1980, the EEA stapler was used to transect the esophagus and obliterate the varices. The procedure is performed through an abdominal incision and is less complicated and more brief than the transthoracic approach. However, there is a problem with rebleeding from gastric varices, and it is not appropriate when the initial hemorrhage is from gastric varices. Again, this is a temporizing procedure.

Angiography

Angiographic procedures have also been utilized for the control of variceal hemorrhage, both with pharmacologic and embolic therapies. Percutaneous transhepatic embolization of varices came into vogue in the mid-1970s. A catheter is introduced into the portal system via the liver; the left and short gastric veins are selectively cannulated and thrombosed with gelatin sponge, autologous clot, or stainless steel coils, close to the origin of the portal vein. This method is a rapid means of obliterating bleeding gastric varices but requires a great deal of interest and skill from the angiographer. The duration of occlusion of varices is unknown, but reappearance of varices has been seen to occur as soon as 3 months after the procedure, with a rebleeding rate of up to 55%. In addition, the complications can be disastrous, including hemorrhage from the hepatic surface, microemboli, bile peritonitis, and portal vein thrombosis (reported to occur in 12% to 36% of cases). Thus, the use of this technique is limited.

Drugs

Pharmacologic therapy has been an option since the early 1960s, when vasopressin was shown to decrease the wedged hepatic venous pressure. Other agents have since been examined as to their usefulness in the treatment of variceal hemorrhage, including somatostatin, nitroglycerin, and propranolol, as well as various analogues of vasopressin. Whereas vasopressin, nitroglycerin, and somatostatin have been used in the treatment of acute hemorrhage, only propranolol has been used in the long-term therapy for either the prophylaxis or prevention of recurrent hemorrhage. Although there are many studies on the use of vasopressin, and its use is widespread, there is not an overwhelming amount of positive evidence as to its absolute efficacy. This goes as well for the analogues of vasopressin, with or without nitroglycerin. Somatostatin has not yet been proved to be ready for wide-scale use in treating variceal hemorrhage. On the other hand, propranolol, though not being utilized during the acute hemorrhage, has been looked at in several studies for preventing recurrent hemorrhage. These studies show contradictory results, leaving the impression that the routine use of propranolol is still experimental. Other agents are being tested for their therapeutic efficacy, and although the hopes for pharmacologic therapy remain high, their routine use at this time is not supported by data. The clinician must still look, then, for a simple, efficacious, and safe method for treating variceal hemorrhage.

Sclerotherapy

Endoscopic injection sclerotherapy may be the answer. Although temporarily abandoned as a therapy for variceal hemorrhage when the portacaval shunt began to be used clinically, a small number of investigators continued to use this method, and in 1974, two reports on 46 patients appeared in the United States. The number of rebleeding episodes appeared to be markedly decreased from what would have been expected. In Great Britain in 1955, Macbeth reported on 30 patients (14 with cirrhosis, 16 with portal or splenic vein thrombosis). Again, however, the enthusiasm for portacaval shunt was so great that injection sclerotherapy faded into the background in both countries. Interest continued to smolder, however, on the European continent over the next several years with small reports. The next large series was not reported until 1973, when Johnston and Rodgers reported on 117 patients and gave a 93% success rate in the control of variceal hemorrhage. The group at Kings College Hospital in London published the first of their many reports on sclerotherapy in 1977. One-year survival in this group of 52 patients was about 58%, but 18% of the deaths were caused by esophageal perforation—most likely caused by the use of the rigid endoscope, rather than the injections themselves.

Though all of these were interesting, it was not until 1975 that the first controlled trial was started by Terblanche and his group in Cape Town. In 1977, the King's College group started a second randomized controlled trial. Their results showed that sclerotherapy reduced the incidence of rebleeding from esophageal varices. However, the study designs were slightly different, as patients in the Cape Town group were allowed to have one additional treatment injection sclerotherapy if they presented with variceal hemorrhage.

The clinician, however, was still hesitant to accept injection sclerotherapy as a treatment of choice, as it involved the rigid endoscope and general anesthesia. Since some thought that part of the problem with shunt surgery was the administration of general anesthesia, there was to be no benefit from sclerotherapy. The introduction of the flexible endoscopes, however, and their utility in injection sclerotherapy has changed this attitude. Most endoscopists who are skilled in esophagogastroduodenoscopy can be trained to perform injection sclerotherapy. Over the years, the number of variations on the theme have been greater almost than the number of centers reporting studies. The rigid endoscope appears almost obsolete, and all studies report the use of flexible endoscopes. Variations still exist: whether an overtube is used to stabilize the esophagus and varices, or whether the "free-hand" method is used. Some investigators prefer a paravariceal injection (i.e., Paquet), where the varices are first occluded by edema and then surrounding fibrosis (similar to the theory for the use of the Sengstaken-Blakemore tube), and others prefer an intravariceal injection, where the varices are directly thrombosed by the sclerosant. However, we have no data comparing intravariceal vs. paravariceal injection. We do know, however, that if a radiopaque solution is mixed with the sclerosant, about 40% of intravariceal injections will be paravariceal. Some investigators will use balloon tamponade of the varices by incorporating a balloon directly onto the endoscope. Tamponade is then applied above the injection site before and during the injection to allow for the engorgement of the varices and the supposed stoppage of outflow of the sclerosant from the immediate site of injection, or over the injection site after the fact, first to stop oozing from the site and also to maintain the sclerosant in the localized area. The number of injections used, the type of injector, and the volume of sclerosant injected have all varied. The most consistent change is that with injections into the paravariceal space, the volume of sclerosant should be small (0.5 to 1.0 ml), whereas intravariceal injection volumes should be higher (2 to 5 ml). The maximum total volume injected appears to be similar, 20 to 30 ml per session.

The solutions that have been used as sclerosants have varied as well: sodium tetradecyl sulfate, sodium morrhuate, ethanolamine oleate, polidocanol, ethanol, TES (a mixture of sodium tetradecyl sulfate, ethanol, and saline), and hypertonic glucose. Some investigators have reported the addition of thrombin or an antibiotic (cephalothin) to the sclerosant. Ethanolamine and polidocanol are not available in the United States, so all studies here use either sodium tetradecyl sulfate or sodium morrhuate in various combinations or percentages. There are only animal studies comparing the efficacy of these solutions, so the choice appears to be up to the endoscopist and the local availability of the solutions. In animal studies by Jensen, both esophageal varices and superficial abdominal wall veins in dogs with portal hypertension were injected with the various sclerosants. It was found that the more efficacious the solution as a sclerosant, the more ulcerogenic it was. Thus, though sodium tetradecyl sulfate and ethanolamine oleate were the best single agents for sclerosis, they showed a 40% incidence of ulcerations. The most well-balanced sclerosant was TES, a 1:1:1 mixture of 3% sodium tetradecyl sulfate, absolute ethanol, and 0.9% saline.

Another variable is the length of time between the injection sessions. It was thought that since the time of highest risk for rebleeding was before the varices were obliterated (which takes an average in most studies of five to six sessions), more frequent injections would decrease the subsequent high-risk bleeding interval. A controlled trial by Westaby et al. compared weekly injections with injections every three weeks. They found that there was a shorter time to achieve obliteration in the patients injected weekly, without a greater number of complications. However, although the early rebleeding rate was not significantly reduced, patients liked weekly injections better, as it allowed them to return to work or complete the therapeutic sessions earlier.

Complications occur in about 12% of patients, or 3.3% of procedures. Minor chest discomfort occurs in 25% to 55%. Fever after sclerotherapy has been noted in up to 50% of patients. The major serious complications include precipitation of bleeding (rare, and controlled with reinjection); esophageal stricture (up to 59%, but averages about 10%); esophageal perforation (1% to 2%); and intramural hematomas. The incidence of strictures appears to be higher in patients receiving paravariceal injections. Although it was feared that there would be cases of acute respiratory failure, as sodium morrhuate produced transient pulmonary hypertension in two patients (which was reproducible in a dog model), this has not appeared to be clinically significant. Less serious complications include the transient chest discomfort, fever, esophageal ulceration (40% to 60% and may be higher depending on the interval between injection sessions), altered esophageal function, chest roentgenographic abnormalities, possible bacteremia, and possible arrhythmias. Complications in this category are minor and should not deter the clinician from subjecting a patient to sclerotherapy. The overall reported mortality is about 1% to 2% of all patients.

Why then should the clinician select sclerotherapy for the patient with bleeding esophageal varices? The published data should be examined in several ways. When compared with a control therapy, (1) Does sclerotherapy better control active bleeding? (2) Does sclerotherapy better control recent bleeding? (3) Does sclerotherapy increase and prolong survival? (4) Does sclerotherapy offer an advantage when compared with the gold standard—shunt surgery—either in survival or cost? (5) Is there any role for prophylactic sclerotherapy?

Active Bleeding

What is the definition of active bleeding? Is there active bleeding, i.e., pumping, spurting, or oozing, from a varix at the time the injection is performed, or merely signs of recent hemorrhage with no other site identified? Although many studies have looked at the use of sclerotherapy in this way, few are well controlled and few address the point of truly "active bleeding." Often, there has been an initial period of vasoconstrictor therapy or balloon tamponade. There are, however, two relevant studies, one from Egypt and one from Germany. The study from Egypt shows a statistically significant control of hemorrhage by sclerotherapy when compared with the Sengstaken-Blakemore tube. The study from Germany, although not showing a significant advantage for sclerotherapy in the initial presenting hemorrhage as compared with standard therapy, does show a significant advantage in control of the rebleeding within that hospitalization. Thus, sclerotherapy is effective acutely, but other methods may control acute bleeding as well.

Recurrent Bleeding

Can recurrent bleeding be controlled and the patient leave the hospital more readily and live longer when treated with sclerotherapy? There are seven published trials of "elective" sclerotherapy vs. "conservative" management. These studies come from King's College Hospital in London, Cape Town, South Africa, Copenhagen, Los Angeles, Egypt, and Germany. In all of these studies, sclerotherapy was compared with "standard" medical therapy. In all of these studies, except for those from Copenhagen and Cape Town, there was a significant decrease in the rebleeding rate over the long-term follow-up period, especially if total obliteration of the varices was achieved. Although the Cape Town study did not show a significant decrease in recurrent hemorrhage, patients in the control arm with a recurrent hemorrhage were allowed to undergo a single session of sclerotherapy. It is not clear how many episodes of bleeding were treated with sclerotherapy in the control group, but since ten of the 14 surviving control group patients had received sclerotherapy during the study, this possibly influenced survival. Although the Copenhagen study did not show a significant difference in the control of the initial hemorrhage, there was a trend in this direction, and 40 days after randomization there was a significant difference in favor of the sclerotherapy group. Thus, it appears that sclerotherapy *does* decrease the rebleeding rate when compared with standard medical therapy.

Survival

Even if the therapy does control the bleeding, what difference does it make to long-term survival? Of the seven studies mentioned above, five have shown a significant increase in survival in the patients treated with sclerotherapy. The most dramatic effect is seen in the study of Paquet and Feussner, where survival is 88% in the sclerotherapy group and 40% in the control patients at 1 year, 68% vs. 22% at 2 years, and 61% vs. 16% at 3 years. Although the Cape Town and Los Angeles studies show no difference between the two groups in survival, the reasons might be that the control group was given an effective additional therapy, mainly emergency sclerotherapy and portacaval shunt, respectively. In a separate analysis, if the patients who had shunt surgery are excluded from both arms of the study, the survival of the sclerotherapy group becomes significant at .05.

A New Gold Standard

Perhaps patients receiving sclerotherapy in these series would have undergone the gold standard of therapy, portacaval shunt, unless they were surgically unfit (too sick or too healthy). Let us compare sclerotherapy with shunt surgery and with pharmacologic therapy. There are several ongoing studies, and two completed and published studies, comparing sclerotherapy with shunt surgery. The first study was performed in San Francisco. Here, 52 patients with Child's class C cirrhosis and variceal hemorrhage requiring 6 or more units of blood were randomized to receive sclerotherapy vs. shunt. In the initial report, presented in 1984, with a mean follow-up period of 263 days, there was no difference in survival between the two groups, although multivariate analysis showed a reduced long-term mortality with sclerotherapy, in a small number of patients, using many variables. The shunt patients initially required more blood, although the sclerotherapy group had more rebleeding during the initial hospitalization and required more days of rehospitalization for rebleeding. However, sclerotherapy was significantly cheaper to perform than surgery. In both groups, 50% died within the initial hospitalization. The authors concluded that since sclerotherapy is as effective as shunt surgery in these severe cirrhotics, and significantly cheaper, it should be the therapy of choice. In a follow-up report, with 64 patients followed up for a mean of 530 days, the duration of the initial hospitalization and the amount of transfusion required was still significantly less in the sclerotherapy group. However, rebleeding from varices, duration of rehospitalization for hemorrhage, and transfusion requirement were all greater in the sclerotherapy group; 40% of these patients required shunt surgery because of recurrent hemorrhage from nonobliterated varices. The authors used an initially aggressive sclerosis protocol but, after discharge, performed sclerotherapy only monthly until obliteration. Several other studies, including the King's College Hospital study, performed sclerotherapy every 1 to 2 weeks until obliteration. Perhaps this is the cause of the need for shunt surgery in such a large proportion of their patients. Because of the high incidence of recurrent hemorrhage, the cost-benefit of sclerotherapy disappeared. However, the authors still thought that because of the high early mortality in the end-stage cirrhotics, and the initial cost-benefits of sclerotherapy, this should still be performed initially, with shunt surgery performed when varices cannot be obliterated or when bleeding continues.

In the second published study (a preliminary report), from Emory University, 71 patients were randomized to receive either sclerotherapy or a distal splenorenal shunt. The population consisted of 56% with Child's class A and B, and 44% with Child's class C disease. In the sclerotherapy group, rebleeding was significantly higher, but in only one third of those who rebled the rebleeding could not be stopped by resclerosis and required surgery. Further, 73% of the patients who "failed" resclerosis were bleeding from either gastritis or gastric varices, conditions not treatable by sclerotherapy. Survival in the sclerotherapy group (including those who went to shunt) was 84% at 2 years, compared with 59% for the shunt group—values significant at .01. Of perhaps even greater importance, hepatic function (as measured by galactose elimination capacity) improved significantly in the sclerotherapy group, even including the patients who failed sclerotherapy and were shunted. The authors, as in the San Francisco study, thought that sclerotherapy should be tried first, with shunt surgery performed when sclerosis failed.

Prophylactic Sclerotherapy

Is there a role for sclerotherapy when varices are seen but no bleeding has occurred? Two published studies show a benefit of this therapy, on both survival and rebleeding. However, in both studies, both the 1-year incidence of bleeding and the 1-year mortality are higher than what would have been expected from the prophylactic portacaval shunt studies performed in the mid-1960s. A preliminary report from King's College Hospital has followed up patients prospectively with varices who have never bled, with no therapy provided. Of 57 patients, ten have bled over a follow-up period of about 24 months. Five of these died, two of whom had Child's grade C cirrhosis and one of whom had a hepatoma. Thus, sclerotherapy performed prophylactically may not have offered a great deal of protection to the entire group. A recent abstract from a VA cooperative study has shown that patients undergoing prophylactic sclerotherapy had a higher rate of rebleeding and complications than the control group. The study was stopped before completion because of this. There are several other studies in progress at present that may further elucidate the role of prophylactic sclerotherapy. Until then, this therapy should remain (in this author's view) within controlled trials.

In conclusion, endoscopic injection sclerotherapy has been shown, in most studies, to decrease the incidence of rebleeding from esophageal varices, especially after the cessation of active hemorrhage (where the data have not been as overwhelming); to prolong survival when compared with standard medical therapy; and to improve or maintain hepatic functional reserve. In the first year after hemorrhage, sclerotherapy is probably also cheaper. It should thus be viewed as the initial therapy in esophageal variceal hemorrhage, with the preliminary data showing that sclerotherapy followed by shunt surgery in the sclerotherapy failures may be the most beneficial road to follow.

Bibliography

1. Barsoum MS, Bolous FI, El-Rooby AA, et al: Tamponade and injection sclerotherapy in the management of bleeding oesophageal varices. *Br J Surg* 1982; 69:76–78.
2. Cello JP, Grendell JH, Crass RA, et al: Endoscopic sclerotherapy versus portacaval shunt in patients with severe cirrhosis and variceal hemorrhage. *N Engl J Med* 1984; 311:1589–1594.
3. Cello JP, Grendell JH, Crass RA, et al: Endoscopic sclerotherapy versus porta caval shunt in patients with severe cirrhosis and acute variceal hemorrhage: Long-term follow-up. *N Engl J Med* 1987; 316:11–15.
4. Copenhagen Esophageal Varices Sclerotherapy Project: Sclerotherapy after first variceal hemorrhage in cirrhosis: A randomized multicenter trial. *N Engl J Med* 1984; 311:1594–1600.
5. Galambos JT: Esophageal variceal hemorrhage: Diagnosis and an overview of treatment. *Semin Liver Dis* 1982; 2:211–226.
6. Korula J, Balart LA, Radvan G, et al: A prospective, randomized controlled trial of chronic esophageal variceal sclerotherapy. *Hepatology* 1985; 5:584–589.
7. MacDougall BRD, Westaby D, Theodossi A, et al: Increased long-term survival in variceal haemorrhage using injection sclerotherapy: Results of a controlled trial. *Lancet* 1982; 1:124–127.
8. Paquet KJ: Prophylactic endoscopic sclerosing treatment of esophageal wall in varices: A prospective controlled randomized trial. *Endoscopy* 1982; 14:4–5.
9. Paquet K–J, Feussner H: Endoscopic sclerosis and esophageal balloon tamponade in acute hemorrhage from esophagogastric varices: A prospective controlled randomized trial. *Hepatology* 1985; 5:580–583.
10. Terblanche J, Bornman PC, Jonker MA, et al: Injection sclerotherapy of esophageal varices. *Semin Liver Dis* 1982; 2:233–241.
11. Terblanche J, Bornman PC, Kahn D, et al: Failure of repeated injection sclerotherapy to improve long-term survival after oesophageal variceal bleeding. *Lancet* 1983; 2:1328–1332.
12. Warren WD, Henderson JM, Millikan WJ, et al: Distal splenorenal shunt versus endoscopic sclerotherapy for long-term management of variceal bleeding: Preliminary report of a prospective, randomized trial. *Ann Surg* 1986; 203:454–462.
13. Westaby D, MacDougall BRD, Williams R: Improved survival following injection sclerotherapy for esophageal varices: Final analysis of a controlled trial. *Hepatology* 1985; 5:827–830.

14. Williams R, Westaby D: Endoscopic sclerotherapy for esophageal varices. *Dig Dis Sci* 1986; 31:108S–121S.
15. Witzel L, Wolbergs E, Merki H: Prophylactic endoscopic sclerotherapy of eosophageal varices: A prospective controlled study. *Lancet* 1981; 1:773–775.
16. Yassin YM, Sherif SM: Randomized controlled trial of injection sclerotherapy for bleeding oesophageal varices: An interim report. *Br J Surg* 1983; 70:20–22.
17. Kern KA, Bower RH, Fischer JE: Surgery for portal hypertension. *Sem Liver Disease* 1982; 2:242–254.

Negative
Richard J. Gusberg, M.D.

Variceal hemorrhage accounts for much of the morbidity and mortality of chronic liver disease associated with portal hypertension. Though only about one third of portal hypertensive cirrhotics ever bleed from their varices, such bleeding is associated with a high rate of recurrence and death.

Though portal pressure elevation and variceal size have been shown to correlate with variceal hemorrhage, there are as yet no reliable and reproducible criteria that can be used to predict with certainty the likelihood of variceal hemorrhage. Because of this, and since the majority of patients with varices will never bleed from them, the therapy directed at variceal bleeding has generally been therapeutic rather than prophylactic: treatment aimed at stopping or preventing bleeding once a variceal hemorrhage has been endoscopically documented.

In the early 1970s, a prospective randomized trial was completed comparing shunts (nonselective) with standard medical therapy in portal hypertensive patients who had not bled from varices. In this study, the shunted patients had poorer short- and long-term survival; clearly, nonselective shunt surgery cannot be considered appropriate prophylaxis. Whether selective shunts or any nonshunt therapies can provide safe and effective proplylaxis for any group of portal hypertensive patients has not been definitively addressed or answered.

Approaches to the treatment of variceal bleeding have been both anatomic and physiologic. Given the underlying hemodynamic problem (increased varix pressure with associated rupture and hemorrhage), the most widely advocated treatment over the last four decades has been aimed at the hemodynamic abnormality: pressure-lowering surgery that shunts blood from the hypertensive portal circulation (portal, splenic, or mesenteric veins) into the lower-pressure systemic system (inferior vena cava or renal veins). These shunts can be either nonselective (i.e., portacaval or mesocaval) or selective (i.e., distal splenorenal or coronary-caval).

Several prospective randomized trials have compared shunt surgery (primary nonselective) with standard supportive therapy in the management of variceal bleeding. Though these trials have certain limitations (e.g., variceal hemorrhage not documented endoscopically, patients predominantly alcoholics from lower socioeconomic groups, data regarding nonbleeding complications not consistently obtained), they represent the best data available that compare shunt surgery with supportive medical therapy. In each of the trials the shunted patients were effectively protected against recurrent variceal bleeding, with a consistent trend favoring longer survival in the shunted patients. When the data from all these trials are combined (done with some justification in view of the comparability of the patient populations and entry criteria), the improved survival following shunt surgery becomes statistically significant. Despite this, the 5-year postshunt survival was no better than 50% to 60%, and shunt surgery represented somewhat of a tradeoff: good control of variceal bleeding but an increased incidence of encephalopathy (though still occurring in the minority of patients) and hepatic failure.

In an effort to preserve the major hemodynamic benefit of nonselective shunts (variceal decompression) and limit the deleterious effects of portal diversion, Warren et al. and Zeppa et al. developed and popularized the selective distal splenorenal shunt (an operation designed to preserve prograde portal flow while still decompressing the varices themselves). Though some patients following selective shunt surgery have progressive loss of prograde portal flow and some series have reported a relatively high incidence of postshunt encephalopathy, the distal splenorenal shunt is generally considered a safe, hemodynamically sound operation that can be performed with a low associated mortality and morbidity: an operation that, when applied appropriately, can provide definitive control of variceal bleeding while minimizing any deleterious effects on hepatic perfusion and function. This appears to be particularly true in patients with nonalcoholic cirrhosis.

Though shunts have been repeatedly demonstrated to be effective in preventing recurrent bleeding, the postoperative development of other, nonbleeding complications has limited the enthusiasm with which they have been advocated and has led to a prolonged search for alternative therapies. Though alcoholic cirrhotic patients, shunted because of variceal bleeding, are unlikely to bleed again from varices, their postshunt course is marked by an increased incidence of portosystemic encephalopathy and eventual death from hepatic failure. The therapy is, therefore, for many patients only palliative, eliminating one of the complications of portal hypertension but neither preventing its other complications nor treating the underlying disturbance in hepatic function. Despite its limitations, however, shunt surgery for bleeding varices remains effective and definitive therapy; in selected patients, it can be performed with a low operative mortality and good long-term survival. Underlying hepatic factors (functional status and histology) are the important determinants of operative and long-term outcomes.

In view of the risks and limitations of shunt surgery, there has been a prolonged search for a better alternative. To be widely recommended as primary treatment, such an alternative should be clearly superior in terms of applicability, effectiveness, risks, or cost. One nonshunt approach that has been recommended widely recently is injection sclerotherapy, a therapeutic procedure that can be performed at the same time as a diagnostic endoscopy. Over the past several years, a considerable sclerotherapy experience has been accumulated. While there are few prospective, randomized trials comparing sclerotherapy with shunt surgery, the accumulated experience has at least begun to define the benefits and risks of this non-operative treatment option. Is sclerotherapy the treatment of choice for all patients with variceal bleeding? The data, both random and randomized, speak for themselves.

Sclerotherapy has been shown to be relatively easy to perform, generally well-tolerated by even sick and unstable patients, often effective at slowing or stopping the bleeding, and relatively inexpensive. The adequate and objective evaluation of the various sclerotherapy trials has, however, been problematic. (1) There has been great variability in the techniques used for sclerotherapy (variability both in the sclerosing agent used and in the timetable of injections). (2) The number of injection sessions required for total variceal obliteration has varied among the series, and the definition of a sclerotherapy failure has been inconsistent (some advocating a position that sclerotherapy not be considered a treatment failure unless variceal bleeding occurs following obliteration of all varices). (3) Since multiple, often uncomfortable, treatment sessions are required before all varices are effectively obliterated, patient compliance is a significant issue (particularly among a largely alcoholic patient population), and although the percentage of noncompliant patients has been said to be as high as 30%, it has been documented poorly in most series. (4) Although varices in the esophagus are generally easy to inject, successful injection and obliteration of gastric varices has not been consistently achievable. (5) Sclerotherapy-related complications have been numerous: esophageal ulcerations and strictures, pulmonary dysfunction, sclerosant escape with splenic venous thrombosis and new or recurrent bleeding. (6) Significant variceal bleeding can occur before variceal obliteration, and recurrent bleeding from gastric or colonic varices following the successful obliteration of the esophageal varices is a recognized problem.

If one therapy is to be recommended as the treatment of choice for all patients with bleeding esophageal varices, it must be shown to be superior to the alternative forms of therapy and widely applicable in patients with cirrhosis of different etiologies and at different stages. The current available data do not support the uniform application of sclerotherapy to cirrhotic patients with variceal hemorrhage.

Despite the apparent ease of applicability of sclerotherapy and the effective control of hemorrhage reported by some authors, no sclerotherapy trial to date has documented an improvement in survival when compared with shunt surgery. A retrospective review of 162 patients treated with sclerotherapy compared with a group treated with supportive medical therapy concluded that the rates of recurrent bleeding and survival were determined by the severity of the underlying liver disease rather than by the therapy chosen. In two prospective, randomized trials comparing sclerotherapy with shunt surgery in patients with variceal bleeding secondary to alcoholic cirrhosis, one showed no treatment benefit among high-risk patients with Child's class C cirrhosis and the other showed a 30% failure to control bleeding in the sclerotherapy group.

Another aspect of the various sclerotherapy trials that has made them difficult to compare has been the different times following hemorrhage at which various treatments have been instituted. In some series, sclerotherapy has been instituted within 24 hours to all patients irrespective of stability or hepatic status; in others, the first course of sclerotherapy was delayed between 1 and 5 days following endoscopic documentation of bleeding, excluding a group of potentially sick and unstable patients with a high likelihood of recurrent bleeding. In addition, the groups that have been studied have not always been comparable in terms of the underlying etiology of the liver disease (alcoholic vs. nonalcoholic) or its complications (e.g., ascites, encephalopathy, hepatic dysfunction).

Furthermore, it will be difficult adequately and objectively to evaluate the therapeutic role of sclerotherapy for variceal bleeding until its techniques become standardized: intravariceal vs. paravariceal injections, type of sclerosing agent, timing of initial injection, timetable for sclerotherapy sessions, and the end point that defines completion of treatment. In addition, the role of sclerotherapy has to be better defined in different treatment groups: emergency vs. elective, alcoholic vs. nonalcoholic, and good risk vs. poor risk.

In poor-risk variceal bleeders with alcoholic cirrhosis, the short- and long-term results of sclerotherapy and shunt surgery are equivalently poor; in good-risk nonalcoholic patients, however, selective shunts are associated with low operative mortality, infrequent recurrent bleeding, and excellent long-term survival (as high as 80% to 90% at 5 years).

It is clear that variceal bleeding is a significant and highly lethal problem for which aggressive therapy is indicated. Despite 40 years of controversy and search for an optimal treatment, no therapy has been identified that is uniformly superior to shunt surgery in all treatment categories. In good-risk (Child's class A) patients with nonalcoholic cirrhosis, the results following distal splenorenal shunt are excellent, with low operative mortality and excellent long-term survival; there is currently no clearly superior nonshunt alternative for this group of patients. In patients with poor hepatic reserve (Child's class C), there is no good evidence that any form of therapy directed at the variceal bleeding alone (either shunt or sclerosis) will effectively alter the otherwise poor prognosis, and the therapies seem to be roughly equivalent in cost. In compliant alcoholic patients of moderate operative risk, who bleed from esophageal rather than gastric varices, and whose bleeding will be predictably controlled by variceal sclerosis (a prediction that cannot currently be made based on the currently available selection criteria), sclerotherapy may be the most effective option.

In summary, shunt surgery is effective and definitive therapy for variceal bleeding and is associated with excellent long-term survival in good-risk nonalcoholic patients. In patients with severe hepatic dysfunction on a nonalcoholic basis, probably the most effective treatment both to prevent recurrent bleeding and to preserve hepatic function is a liver transplant. In the poor-risk alcoholic patient (notoriously noncompliant), a shunt operation may provide more effective long-term control at no increased cost. Whether sclerotherapy is the treatment of choice for any moderate-risk patient bleeding from varices cannot be definitively determined until the techniques and applications of sclerotherapy have been better standardized and defined, with the outcomes more accurately predicted before treatment. Until that time, sclerotherapy seems to have more utility as a temporizing tool or a secondary treatment option than as definitive primary therapy for all variceal bleeders.

The major therapeutic challenge for patients with bleeding varices remains incompletely answered: How can we appropriately select particular therapies for particular patients? Until we have criteria that can be reproducibly utilized to predict posttreatment outcomes, shunt surgery should remain the superior standard against which all others must be judged. Is sclerotherapy the treatment of choice for patients with bleeding varices? Yes for a few, no for many, and maybe for the rest. Though sclerotherapy can be effective treatment in selected groups of patients, the criteria that can effectively guide such selection remain obscure. Until such criteria are firmly established, it will remain a treatment looking for a clear and supportable indication.

Bibliography

1. Cello JP, Grendell JOH, Crass RA, et al: Endoscopic sclerotherapy versus portacaval shunt in patients with severe cirrhosis and acute variceal hemorrhage. *N Engl J Med* 1987; 316:11–15.
2. DiMagno EP, Zinsmeister AR, Larson DE, et al: Influence of hepatic reserve and cause of esophageal varices on survival and rebleeding before and after the introduction of sclerotherapy: A retrospective analysis. *Mayo Clin Proc* 1985; 60:149–157.
3. Langer B, Taylor BR, MacKenzie T, et al: Further report of a prospective randomized trial comparing distal splenorenal shunt with end-to-side portacaval shunt. *Gastroenterology* 1985; 88:424–429.
4. Rekkers LF, Rudman D, Galambos JT, et al: A randomized, controlled trial of the distal splenorenal shunt. *Ann Surg* 1977; 188:271–282.
5. Warren WD, Henderson TM, Millikan WJ, et al: Distal splenorenal shunt versus endoscopic sclerotherapy for long-term management of variceal bleeding. *Ann Surg* 1986; 203:454–462.
6. Zeppa R, Hensley GT, Levi JV, et al: The comparative survivals of alcoholics vs. non-alcoholics after distal splenorenal shunt. *Ann Surg* 1978; 187:510–513.

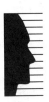

Rebuttal: Affirmative
Rosemarie Fisher, M.D.

In the preceding commentary opposing the view that sclerotherapy is the initial choice for treating variceal hemorrhage, the author answers "yes for a few, no for many, and maybe for the rest." However, the data presented in the initial positive statement, and the data presented by himself, would change that statement to no for a few, yes for many, and maybe for the rest. As was stated initially, the major problems in supporting sclerotherapy for "the many" lie with the variety of the studies presented, including the timing of sclerosis after a hemorrhage; the type of injection used (intravariceal or paravariceal); the sclerosant used; the underlying cause of the liver disease; the timetable for sclerotherapy sessions; the definition of failure of therapy; and the lack of large studies comparing sclerotherapy with shunt surgery.

Yes, some patients are not candidates for sclerotherapy. Such patients need to be directed toward other therapies, e.g., shunt surgery. Some are readily identified: the patient bleeding from gastric varices, where the rebleeding rate after sclerotherapy has been extremely high; the patient who rebleeds every few days in the hospital while undergoing sclerotherapy; the patient who cannot tolerate multiple endoscopies. We need to define the criteria that will allow us to decide at the time of the index variceal hemorrhage whether the individual patient will not respond to sclerotherapy and should be sent to shunt surgery. Until such criteria are established, however, the number of patients in whom sclerotherapy is contraindicated, or in whom it will be known to fail, is small.

The timing of therapy initiation after variceal hemorrhage is highly variable in the published reports on both sclerotherapy and shunt surgery. The optimal timing of therapy needs to be better defined. With sclerotherapy, there may be no critical timing: whenever it is initiated in the immediate perihemorrhage period, it will prevent recurrent acute hemorrhage in most patients.

The question about the type of injection used, either intravariceal or paravariceal, does not appear to be a major issue. Although various authors stoutly support their own method, studies have shown that up to 40% of the intended intravariceal injections will be paravariceal, and the reverse is also likely to a smaller extent. Thus, neither method is pure, yet they both stop hemorrhage.

The timing of the sclerosing sessions has not appeared to make a major difference in the studies performed thus far. In the study by Williams and Westaby, patients were randomized to 1-week or 3-week intervals between injection sessions. They showed no difference in the frequency of early rebleeding between the two groups but did show an earlier time of obliteration of varices in the more frequently injected group and an earlier time of return to work. The main point is to avoid long periods between sessions—the sooner the varices can be obliterated, the better. This would also tend to increase the compliance of the alcoholic population who might otherwise be lost to follow-up.

The stratification of patients by type of underlying liver disease is not a problem new to sclerotherapy. This problem has long plagued the shunt studies. The problem will remain, however, as long as alcoholic cirrhosis remains the major cause of liver disease in this country. The randomization of patients with nonalcoholic liver disease to either shunt surgery or sclerotherapy, though needed and important, will be difficult unless multicenter studies are performed that will enable the enrollment of large numbers of patients.

The information available on the complications of sclerotherapy stand as presented—they are frequent but rarely severe and are easily treated. The initial data on pulmonary complications of sclerotherapy have not been substantiated. There is thus far no documented proof of rebleeding from gastric or colonic varices after successful obliteration of esophageal varices.

The end point of sclerotherapy is clear: obliteration of all esophageal varices. The definition of a sclerotherapy failure remains somewhat ethical. However, this can be decided in the individual institution and the individual patient, even before the start of therapy.

It should also be remembered that not every patient is a candidate for shunt surgery. Though most of this group involves the poor-risk, Child's class C cirrhotic patient, there are also others—those with splenic and portal vein thrombosis, those with small renal veins (when splenorenal shunts are planned), and those whose operative mortality is high based on other medical problems.

Still to be mentioned is one additional group where sclerotherapy is preferable to shunt surgery: the pediatric population. As the child grows, the shunt might not provide long-term efficacy. Transplantation may be the best alternative, and if so, both the physician and surgeon will prefer to have avoided previous surgery on the portal system.

It still remains for several large-scale studies to answer a large proportion of the above questions. However, the early results of studies comparing shunt surgery to sclerotherapy (including the one by Warren et al. from Atlanta) support the notion that sclerotherapy initially will stop and prevent variceal hemorrhage in the majority of patients. During this process there is improvement in hepatic functional capacity. Failures of sclerotherapy that are then subsequently treated by shunt surgery appear to do extremely well. Perhaps, then, the preferred route of therapy will be sclerotherapy initially, allowing stabilization of the patient and improvement of hepatic function, a solid definition of failure of sclerotherapy (agreed on at the start of therapy by both the surgeon and the endoscopist), followed by shunt surgery in those patients who fail sclerotherapy. The long-term results of such studies are eagerly awaited. Perhaps then the debate may be settled.

Until then, however, one important point needs to be made in conclusion. Sclerotherapy has been shown to be effective in stopping variceal hemorrhage and preventing the recurrence of hemorrhage in a large proportion of patients in many published studies. It is a comparatively safe procedure, performed by most trained endoscopists, and readily available at most institutions. It is a treatment option with a clear and supportable indication—esophageal variceal hemorrhage. Distal splenorenal shunt, although not clearly better than portacaval shunt, appears to be the shunt of choice in most patients, especially those with nonalcoholic liver disease. It is not anatomically possible in all patients. Not all surgeons performing shunt surgery are capable of, or comfortable with, performing distal splenorenal shunt, nor do they have high long-term rates of shunt patency and low rebleeding rates.

Thus, until we have definitive data on the comparison of shunt surgery vs. sclerotherapy in large, long-term studies, and until every hospital has an outstanding vascular surgeon on its staff, sclerotherapy is the initial (even if temporizing) therapy of choice in most cirrhotic patients presenting with esophageal variceal hemorrhage.

Bibliography

1. Warren WD, Henderson JM, Millikan WJ, et al: Distal splenorenal shunt versus endoscopic sclerotherapy for long-term management of variceal bleeding: Preliminary report of a prospective, randomized trial. *Ann Surg* 1986; 203:454–462.
2. Williams R, Westaby D: Endoscopic sclerotherapy for esophageal varices. *Dig Dis Sci* 1986; 31:1085–1215.

Rebuttal: Negative
Richard J. Gusberg, M.D.

In view of the morbidity and mortality of variceal hemorrhage, one documented episode of variceal bleeding mandates a treatment plan aimed to prevent its recurrence. Treatment stages can be characterized by (1) immediate control, (2) optimization of status, and (3) definitive therapy. There are multiple therapies available to prevent or control variceal bleeding. Furthermore, the problems and prognosis of portal hypertension and variceal bleeding vary in relation to the underlying anatomic, metabolic, and hemodynamic derangements. The challenge is to match the most appropriate therapy to the particular patient. The real question is not whether a treatment is indicated but when it can be utilized most effectively.

Sclerotherapy is relatively safe and often effective—under certain circumstances. Until its techniques become standardized and appropriate randomized trials with sufficient follow-up are completed, its broad applicability will remain based on anecdotal, uncontrolled, or uncertain data. As a treatment that doesn't address the underlying hemodynamic abnormality, persistently elevated portal pressure and recurrent bleeding characterize the late follow-up of patients undergoing sclerotherapy. In addition, sclerosant escape and partial splanchnic venous thrombosis may limit the operative decompression options. Complications of the sclerotherapy, uninjectable gastric varices, noncompliance, between-treatment variceal hemorrhage, bleeding-precipitated hospital admissions that increase with time following sclerotherapy (associated with increasing cost of care), and no definitive evidence from prospective trials that sclerotherapy can provide any survival advantage when compared with shunt surgery all raise serious questions as to the rationale for its uniform, widespread applicability. It is the minority of sclerotherapy patients whose posttreatment course is marked by compliance, no complications, and definitive control of bleeding. The most appropriate role for sclerotherapy would seem to be initial control and stabilization in patients bleeding from esophageal (rather than gastric) varices and long-term control in selected, compliant patients who are considered inappropriate surgical candidates. When performed appropriately, in appropriately selected patients, shunt surgery remains a safe, definitive, and effective therapy.

It seems clear that in the overall management of cirrhotic, portal hypertensive patients with variceal bleeding, some patients merit sclerotherapy, some patients merit shunt surgery, and in some patients the appropriate therapy is a transplant. All these treatment modalities are effective in selected patients; none of these treatments can be uniformly recommended for all patients with variceal bleeding. The real therapeutic challenge lies in the identification of the criteria that can allow us appropriately to match the patient to the treatment.

Editor's Comments
Thomas P. Duffy, M.D.

No cure exists for reversal of the cirrhotic lesion in liver disease short of the major, threatening undertaking of organ transplantation. But even before end-stage liver disease, the life of the cirrhotic patient may be abbreviated by sudden esophageal bleeding, an event that represents a mechanical failure due to elevation in the portal pressure secondary to obstruction in the hepatic circuit. The vagaries that determine when such an eruption will occur are so many and so ill understood that successful means of prophylactic treatment in preventing esophageal bleeding still elude both the internist and surgeon.

Dr. Gusberg has forcefully iterated the positive outcome that can be purchased with the "gold standard" of selective shunt surgery for bleeding esophageal varices. The multiple other routes of intervention outlined by Dr. Fisher (angiography, drugs, sclerotherapy) suggest that the gold standard is not the immediate or available choice for most physicians. Shunt procedures require prolonged operating times with the compounded insult of anesthesia to the already damaged liver. Freedom from the need of general anesthesia makes sclerotherapy an important alternative to shunt surgery in these patients with advanced hepatic disease.

Admittedly, sclerotherapy suffers from a problem with its image; it is a technique that puts out brush fires but does nothing about their cause. Shunt surgery has a modicum of appeal because it corrects the abnormal, heightened pressure that creates the esophageal varix. In those circumstances where the mechanical problem is foremost (vascular obstruction without significant hepatocellular disease), shunt surgery may almost be curative. However, the majority of cirrhotic livers are the aftermath of intrinsic hepatocellular disease, and in these patients, shunt surgery is also only a means of putting out brush fires.

There does not seem to be an adequate basis in the data provided to assign absolute territorial rights to either sclerotherapy or shunt surgery. Anyone who experienced the futility and difficulties in using the Sengstaken-Blakemore tube is pleased to have sclerotherapy as a legitimate option to stay esophageal bleeding. With the fires contained, choosing candidates appropriate for surgery and preparing them for surgery are welcome tasks in the management of these patients. The claims for either treatment should not be too enthusiastic or uncritical; they are both means to eliminate or stall the signs of underlying organ dysfunction. Ongoing studies should permit their proper allocation in the difficult problem of esophageal variceal bleeding.

Some Patients With Chronic Active Hepatitis B Should Be Treated With Corticosteroids

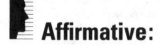

Chapter Editor: Gary Gitnick, M.D.

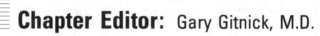

Affirmative: Evangelista Sagnelli, M.D.
Associate Professor of Clinical Virology,
Clinic of Infectious Diseases, First School of
Medicine, University of Naples, Naples, Italy

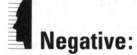

Negative: Gary L. Davis, M.D.
Associate Professor of Medicine, Division of
Gastroenterology, Hepatology and Nutrition,
University of Florida, College of Medicine,
Gainesville, Florida

Debates in Medicine 1:86–117, 1988
©1988, Year Book Medical Publishers, Inc.
0887-218X/88/01-86-117-$04.00

Affirmative
Evangelista Sagnelli, M.D.

In treating patients with hepatitis B surface antigen (HB$_s$Ag)–positive chronic active hepatitis (CAH), the rationale for using corticosteroids, alone or in combination with azathioprine, is based on the observation that this treatment may inhibit the interaction between sensitized T lymphocytes and viral antigens or autoantigens expressed on the membranes of the hepatocytes.[1] The prevention of lymphocyte cytotoxic reaction may reduce liver cell necrosis and consequently clinical symptoms and biochemical alteration. On the other hand, corticosteroids enhance hepatitis B virus (HBV) replication[2, 3] either because of the inhibited cytotoxic activity of T lymphocytes with a consequent increase in the number of infected hepatocytes or because of a direct action on HBV synthesis in the liver cells. Before this rationale was formulated, some authors started treating patients with HB$_s$Ag-positive CAH with corticosteroids only, because these drugs had been demonstrated effective in autoimmune CAH, a disease with liver histology similar to that of HB$_s$Ag-positive CAH.[4–6] Unfortunately, early studies reported that corticosteroids were less effective in HB$_s$Ag-positive CAH than in autoimmune CAH. However, a high percentage of patients with symptomatic active cirrhosis were included in these studies, and only a limited number of patients were HB$_s$Ag positive.

Further available reports are either limited or nonrandomized, and the results are conflicting. Whereas some authors reported moderate benefit or no effectiveness whatsoever or even deleterious effects, others published more optimistic data. In nonrandomized studies (which, however, included a great number of patients), Tsuji et al.[10] in Japan and Giusti et al.[16] in Italy observed that prednisone, given alone or in combination with azathioprine, may favorably modify the clinical course of HB$_s$Ag-positive CAH, even if the development of cirrhosis is not prevented. On the other hand, Lam et al.[11] in Hong Kong in a controlled randomized trial carried out on a limited number of patients observed deleterious effects of prednisolone. This was the first of many studies carried out from 1971 to 1981 that reported harmful effects of corticosteroids on HB$_s$Ag-positive CAH. Indeed, such deleterious effects have been shown by actuarial survival rate analysis, but by the end of the study death had occurred in seven of the 25 patients receiving prednisolone and also in eight of the 26 untreated patients. Moreover, more than 40% of patients included in this study had morphologic evidence of cirrhosis that in some might have been inactive, as shown by the normal aminotransferase values observed by Lam et al. in some patients at the time they entered the study. It should also be noted that most of the patients studied by Lam et al. showed symptoms, whereas most patients with HB$_s$Ag-positive CAH generally become symptomatic only in the advanced phase of the disease. Overall, it is my opinion that the data of Lam et al. suggest a harmful effect of corticosteroids only in symptomatic patients with established cirrhosis and that no generalization can be made for all patients with HB$_s$Ag-positive CAH.

Other investigators have reported that corticosteroids may be of moderate benefit or ineffective. Schalm et al.[7] observed that patients with HB$_s$Ag-positive CAH infrequently showed remission when treated with conventional doses of corticosteroids (20 mg/day), whereas with higher doses (60 mg/day) improvement was more frequently found. No effectiveness was observed by Smith et al.[12] in the United States and by Mayer zum Buschenfelde et al.[9] in Berlin in nonrandomized studies.

It is surprising that so many clinical studies carried out in qualified liver units should give such conflicting results. Indeed, on reviewing these studies, it appears that different principles were used either for selecting patients or for evaluating the course of the disease. Moreover, there were differences in treatment schedules, in the ethnic background of patients, and in the percentages of male homosexuals, drug abusers, patients with liver cirrhosis, those with history of alcoholic intake, those with HBV active replication and possibly those with superinfection from hepatitis delta virus (HDV) or non-A, non-B viruses. Therefore, we must admit that after 15 years of investigations it is still unknown whether corticosteroids are useful for patients with HB$_s$Ag-positive CAH. The only truth emerging from this entangled state of conflicting data is that corticosteroids are of benefit only to some patients with HB$_s$Ag-positive CAH. Of course, the problem is how these patients are to be identified before starting treatment.

In 1983 we published the results of our prospective study, which analyzed the effect of immunosuppressive therapy on HB$_s$Ag-positive CAH in relation to the presence or absence of HB$_e$Ag and anti-HB$_e$.[16] We treated 51 patients with 100 mg of azathioprine daily, 51 with 20 mg of prednisolone daily, 51 with a combination of 20 mg of prednisolone and 50 mg of azathioprine daily, and left 51 patients untreated. The results were evaluated at the time of a second liver biopsy, after 2 years of observation, on the bases of a physical examination, serum liver tests, and liver histologic study. None of the treatments proved to be beneficial to HB$_e$Ag-positive patients, whereas HB$_e$Ag-negative patients responded favorably only to the combination of prednisolone and azathioprine. In fact, HB$_e$Ag-negative patients treated with the combination of the two drugs, as compared with the untreated ones, more frequently showed a clear reduction in both serum aminotransferase values and in the entity of piecemeal necrosis and less frequently developed cirrhosis. Moreover, among anti-HB$_e$–positive patients, improvement was observed in 16 (59%) of the 27 patients receiving prednisolone plus azathioprine but in only three (13%) of the 23 untreated patients. Since HBV replication is active in HB$_e$Ag-positive patients and absent or reduced to low levels in anti-HB$_e$–positive ones, and is enhanced by immunosuppressive therapy,[2, 3] the possibility exists that active viral replication may limit the effectiveness of this therapy. Since 10% to 30% of anti-HB$_e$–positive patients show a detectable amount of circulating Dane particles, as detected by the presence of HBV DNA in serum, the influence of HBV replication on the response to treatment could be better evaluated by determining the presence of HBV DNA rather than the HB$_e$Ag/anti-HB$_e$ system.

What is the reason for HBV replication inhibiting the response to immunosuppressive therapy? Proof has been given by in vitro cytotoxicity experiments that the core antigen (HB$_c$Ag) present on the membranes of hepatocytes is a target, or at least one of the targets, for T cell cytotoxic activity, which perpetuates the liver damage, giving the histologic lesions characteristic of CAH (parenchymal necrosis, piecemeal necrosis, lymphomonocytic cell infiltration).[19] Immunosuppressive therapy, by enhancing HBV replication, may determine an increased expression of HB$_c$Ag on the membranes of hepatocytes with a consequent increase in the T cell–mediated cytotoxicity. It is my opinion, however, that these observations do not give an exhaustive answer to the question. Moreover, HBV replication is not the only factor influencing the response to immunosuppressive therapy. In fact, the combination of prednisolone and azathioprine favorably influenced the course of the disease only in 46% of our anti-HB$_e$–positive patients.

The stage of the disease is another factor to be taken into consideration before treating patients with HB$_s$Ag-positive CAH. As mentioned before, patients with established cirrhosis should not be treated with corticosteroids.

Patients with mild CAH without cirrhosis were investigated by Romeo et al.[13] in Italy in a randomized study. Twenty-two corticosteroid-treated patients received a dosage of 20 mg daily of prednisolone, reduced to 10 mg daily 2 months after the normalization of serum liver tests; the treatment was discontinued 3 months after clinical, biochemical, and histologic remission. How long these patients were treated remains unclear. After 3 months of follow-up, patients treated with corticosteroids showed remission more frequently than the 22 patients in the placebo-treated group. Then, possibly due to the lowered dosage of prednisolone, the beneficial effects of the corticosteroids were no longer evident, and after discontinuation of therapy relapses occurred more frequently in treated patients than in the placebo group ($P < .001$). Subsequently, treated patients developed cirrhosis more frequently than those untreated (50% vs. 4.5%). The data of this study seem to indicate than, rather than corticosteroids, discontinuation of therapy may be deleterious for patients with HB$_s$Ag-positive mild CAH.

Whether these patients should receive treatment is still doubtful. During 1 year of follow-up, the untreated patients in Romeo's study frequently showed remission (36.3%), infrequently had relapses (9%), and rarely developed cirrhosis (4.5%). Instead, progression to cirrhosis was observed in

12 (71%) of 17 patients treated with corticosteroids by De Groote et al.[8] in Belgium; this study, however, did not include untreated patients. These observations suggest that patients with mild CAH should be left untreated until more effective drugs become available.

Patients with severe CAH without morphologic evidence of cirrhosis should receive treatment since they frequently progress to cirrhosis. Of 22 untreated anti-HB$_e$–positive patients with severe CAH observed in our liver unit, seven (32%) developed cirrhosis after 2 years and 12 (55%) after 4 years of observation. These rates were lower in the 24 anti-HB$_e$–positive patients treated with the association of prednisolone and azathioprine, 8% after 2 years and 25% after 4 years.

Thus, immunosuppressive therapy should be considered only for HBV DNA-negative patients without established cirrhosis and with liver histology showing severe activity (bridging necrosis, multilobular necrosis, or wide piecemeal necrosis). However, "the exception proves the rule," as an Italian saying goes, and proverbs contain the wisdom of the people. In fact, I have observed a few symptomatic patients with severe CAH, some of them with cirrhosis, and active HBV replication who improved with corticosteroids given in combination with azathioprine and in one case with azathioprine alone. I would like to report two of these cases, because it is my opinion that we should learn not only from double-blind trials but also from the individual cases we observe day by day in our wards and in our private practices.

Case 1

A 14-year-old boy was admitted to our liver unit in May 1977 with HB$_s$-antigenemia and increased aminotransferase values over the previous 10 months (Fig 1). A liver biopsy performed at the time of hospitalization showed CAH with severe activity without cirrhosis. The bilirubin level was normal, and alanine aminotransferase (ALT) and γ-globulin values were high (ALT, nine times the maximum normal value; γ-globulins, 2.4 gm/dl). Serum markers of HBV replication were performed later on a serum sample stored at $-20°C$; this boy was HB$_e$Ag positive, HBV DNA positive, and Dane-HB$_c$Ag positive on starting treatment with prednisolone, 20 mg, and azathioprine, 50 mg daily. Moreover, he was hepatitis delta antigen (HDAg) positive on the first liver biopsy. The ALT values dropped during treatment, and two relapses occurred when the patient abruptly discontinued therapy after 6 and 18 months. Relapses were mild and characterized only by an increase in serum ALT values. Treatment was readily restored, and a clear reduction in ALT values was obtained on both occasions. After 32 months of therapy, I decided to reduce the dosage of prednisolone to 10 mg/day because the patient had developed moderate obesity and also

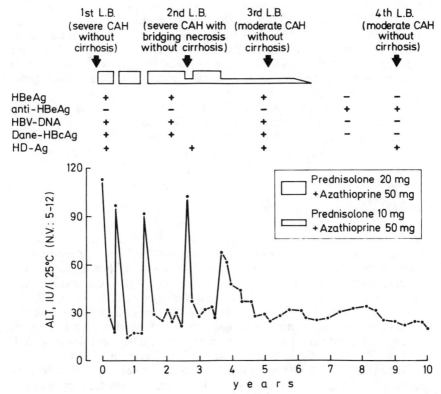

FIG 1.
Course of the disease in a 14-year-old boy with hepatitis B e antigen (HB$_e$Ag)–positive severe chronic active hepatitis *(CAH),* treated with prednisolone and aza-thioprine. *HBV* indicates hepatitis B virus; *HDAg,* hepatitis delta antigen; *L.B.,* liver biopsy; *ALT,* alanine aminotransferase; *N.V.,* normal value.

because the time had come to start a tapered discontinuation of therapy. At the same time, a second liver biopsy was suggested. This biopsy was performed 30 days after the reduction in the dosage of prednisolone, i.e., at the time of a third relapse similar to those observed previously. The second liver biopsy showed severe CAH with a few bridges of necrosis, without evidence of cirrhosis; HDAg was still present. The initial treatment was then restored and administered for 8 months. A subsequent reduction in the prednisolone dosage to 10 mg was followed only by a transitory moderate increase in ALT values. The treatment with 10 mg of predniso-lone and 50 mg of azathioprine daily was given for 15 months, then sub-sequently tapered and finally discontinued. A third liver biopsy was performed after 5 years of observation and a fourth one after 9 years. Both showed CAH of moderate activity without bridging necrosis and without cirrhosis; HDAg was detected in both biopsies. After discontinuation of therapy, seroconversion to anti-HB$_e$ was observed, and HBV DNA and Dane-HB$_c$Ag became undetectable. After 10 years of observation the boy had become a diligent student in excellent clinical condition. This, I think, was an excellent result.

I have learned a lot from this case. First, immunosuppressive therapy may be effective even in some patients with HBV replication. Second, mild relapses may not have deleterious effects. Third, persistence of HDV infection does not impair the response to immunosuppressive treatment.

Case 2

A 34-year-old man was hospitalized in June 1979 with jaundice (Fig 2). He had diabetes requiring insulin treatment and had had HB$_s$Ag-positive chronic liver disease for at least 2 years. At the time of hospitalization the patient was icteric, symptomatic, and HB$_s$Ag-, HB$_e$Ag-, and Dane-HB$_c$Ag– positive in a serum sample obtained on admittance and stored at $-20°C$. In this serum sample, HBV DNA was subsequently detected, whereas antibodies to HDAg were absent. A liver biopsy showed severe CAH with cirrhosis and widespread parenchymal necrosis; HDAg was not detected. Since his clinical condition deteriorated and ALT and bilirubin levels were persistently high (ALT, 40 times the maximum normal value; bilirubin, 24 mg/dl), something had to be done. At that time, antiviral therapy was not available, and the patient had diabetes, which contraindicates corticosteroid administration. I started treating this patient with 100 mg of azathioprine daily, hoping for an improvement in his clinical condition. Surprisingly, his clinical condition improved rapidly and the patient became asymptomatic and anicteric after 35 days of treatment. The ALT values also dropped. This treatment was continued for about 2 years, after which the dosage of azathioprine was reduced to 50 mg for another 2 years and then discontinued. A second liver biopsy performed at that time showed cirrhosis with mild inflammatory activity and no sign of HDV infection. After the discontinuation of therapy, seroconversion to anti-HB$_e$ was observed. Both HBV DNA and Dane-HB$_c$Ag became undetectable. No relapses or complications in the cirrhosis or side effects of treatment were observed. After 7 years of observation, this patient is still HB$_s$Ag positive and in good clinical condition.

I do not know whether the improvement after the administration of azathioprine would have come about even if the patient had been left untreated. It has been demonstrated that azathioprine administered alone is not effective in HB$_s$Ag-positive CAH and its use should be discouraged.

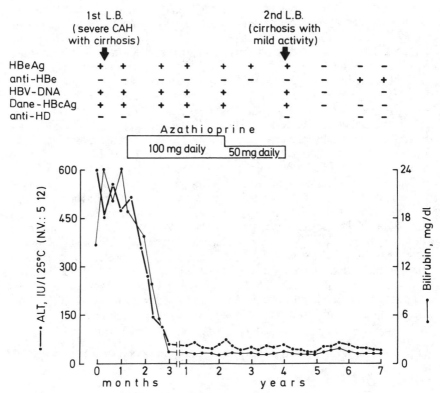

FIG 2.
Course of the disease in a 34-year-old man with hepatitis B e antigen (HB$_e$Ag)–positive severe chronic active hepatitis (CAH) with cirrhosis, treated only with azathioprine because of diabetes requiring insulin. *L.B.* indicates liver biopsy; *HBV,* hepatitis B virus; *HD,* hepatitis delta virus; *ALT,* alanine aminotransferase; *N.V.,* normal value.

This treatment was used for this patient as an *extrema ratio*. On the whole, I think that this patient was simply lucky.

Influence of HDV Infection on the Course of the Disease and the Response to Corticosteroids

Patients with HB$_s$Ag-positive CAH who have HDV infection show an unfavorable outcome more frequently than those without this infection.[14]

I observed 45 consecutive patients with HB$_s$Ag-positive CAH without cirrhosis each for a period of at least 2 years.[17] The patients were treated at
random with 15 mg of prednisolone or left untreated. On the first liver
biopsy, HDAg was detected in 33 (73%) of the 45 patients. Among these
33 HDAg-positive patients, three (19%) of the 16 who were treated and
six (35%) of those 17 left untreated had become HDAg negative by the
second liver biopsy. After 2 years of observation, development of cirrhosis
was observed in 38% of patients with persistent HDV replication and in
5% of the patients who were clear of HDV or had never had HDAg; no
differences were observed between treated and untreated patients. Thus,
prednisolone at a dosage of 15 mg daily did not modify the course of the
disease either in HDAg-positive or in HDAg-negative patients. However,
in another clinical study we carried out, the combination of 20 mg of prednisolone and 50 mg of azathioprine was shown to be helpful for anti-HB$_e$–
positive patients whether HDAg-positive or HDAg-negative. Of the 24
treated anti-HB$_e$–positive patients, deterioration was observed in three
(17%) of the 18 HDAg-positive patients and in none of the 6 HDAg-negative ones, whereas among 25 untreated anti-HB$_e$–positive patients, an
unfavorable outcome was seen in 11 (65%) of the 17 HDAg-positive and
in one (16%) of the eight HDAg-negative patients. These observations
suggest that HDV infection does not modify the response to immunosuppressive therapy and that the dosage of drugs may be important.

The Influence of Relapses on the Clinical Course of CAH

A sudden discontinuation of corticosteroids is followed by an increase in
aminotransferase levels in about 50% of cases during the following 6
months, and in some patients clinical symptoms may reappear, indicating
an exacerbation of the disease. In most cases this exacerbation is moderate
and followed by remission, but in some cases it has led to severe and even
fatal hepatitis.[20, 21] Thus, for the greater part of patients with HB$_s$Ag-posi-
tive CAH who show a relapse, it may be an error to restart corticosteroid
treatment since another relapse may occur when therapy is again discontinued. I think that frequent relapses over a short period may be harmful
for these patients (case 1 reported above is an exception). This opinion,
however, is not based on data from clinical trials but on my own clinical
practice on hundreds of HB$_s$Ag-positive patients with CAH, some of whom
discontinued corticosteroid therapy by themselves and came to the physician once a relapse had occurred. Thus, even the reliability of patients
should be taken into consideration before treating them with corticosteroids.

On the whole, relapses should be avoided or at least limited. In my experience, a gradual breaking off of immunosuppressive therapy may reduce the occurrence and limit the frequency of relapses. However, no prospective study on this topic has been carried out.

Side Effects of Therapy

Side effects occur frequently during long-term administration of corticosteroids. This has been clearly shown in a multicenter retrospective study, coordinated by Giusti in Italy, on 867 patients with chronic hepatitis observed in 12 liver units for periods ranging from 1 to 10 years. Of these patients, 473 were HB$_s$Ag positive.[15] Severe side effects (diabetes, peptic ulcer, tuberculosis, arterial hypertension, osteoporosis, etc.), which in most cases impede continuing therapy, occurred in 15.3% of the 529 patients receiving corticosteroids alone or in combination with azathioprine and in 4.4% of the 253 untreated patients. Leukocytopenia or thrombocytopenia occurred in 8.2% of the 85 patients treated with azathioprine alone and in 4.6% of the 242 patients receiving this drug in combination with corticosteroids. Thus, more than 80% of patients with CAH develop no side effects requiring the discontinuation of therapy.

Final Considerations

Immunosuppressive therapy may be taken into consideration for treating some patients with HB$_s$Ag-positive CAH, since no other drug has proved capable of favorably modifying the course of the disease. Patients who may improve with corticosteroids given in association with azathioprine are those with severe histologic lesions, either symptomatic or asymptomatic, without established cirrhosis and with the absence of markers of HBV replication in serum. To give an idea of the numbers, I can only answer that such patients amount to about 20% of all HB$_s$Ag-positive patients with CAH observed in our liver unit, and that this percentage may vary from one liver unit to another, thus reflecting the different manners of grouping patients.

In my experience, long-term treatment with 15 or 20 mg of prednisolone daily did not modify the course of the disease, whereas the combination of 20 mg of prednisolone and 50 mg of azathioprine daily showed a fairly good effect on anti-HB$_e$–positive patients. Of course, by increasing the dosage of immunosuppressive drugs, greater immunosuppression may be obtained, but severe side effects may occur more frequently. Thus, this treatment should be given only to selected patients, but at a dosage that may be effective regardless of the presence or absence of HDV infection. Of course, I do not think that all HB$_s$Ag/HBV DNA-negative patients with severe progressive CAH and without established cirrhosis would respond favorably to immunosuppressive therapy. I share the idea of Sherlock and Thomas[18] that patients with the conditions mentioned above may be treated with a combination of corticosteroids and azathioprine for 2 to 3 months and carefully observed during treatment to evaluate whether any clinical and/or biochemical improvement occurs. Treatment should be gradually discontinued in patients showing deterioration or no change, and continued for 18 to 24 months in those showing improvement. After 2 years of treatment, azathioprine should be discontinued and prednisolone gradually tapered to reduce the risk of relapses. Of course, the appearance of serious side effects excludes the continuation of treatment.

Treatment schedules, data, and opinions reported herein refer only to the adult population of HB$_s$Ag-positive patients with CAH. Very little is known on the effectiveness of corticosteroids in children with HB$_s$Ag-positive CAH. Conflicting data come from three available studies, all carried out in Italy, which are either too limited or nonrandomized. Corticosteroids are reported as beneficial by Tolentino et al.[22] in Genoa, ineffective by Vajro et al.[23] in Naples, and deleterious by Maggiore et al.[24] in Milan. Again, differences in the treatment schedules, in the selection of patients, and in the criteria to evaluate the outcome make a conclusive evaluation of the efficacy of corticosteroids impossible in children with HB$_s$Ag-positive CAH. However, children infrequently show severe CAH and are frequently HB$_e$Ag positive. Thus, I think that this therapy should only occasionally be taken into consideration for treating children with HB$_s$Ag-positive CAH.

Acknowledgment

I wish to thank the director of my institute, Prof. Giuseppe Giusti, and my friends Prof. Felice Piccinino and Prof. Giuseppe Manzillo, for the opportunity they have given me to reexamine the case histories of patients with CAH they have followed up for years. I wish also to acknowledge the expert assistance of my coworkers Dr. F. M. Felaco, Dr. P. Filippini, Dr. G. Pasquale, and Dr. P. Peinetti, and the technical assistance of Dr. E. Buonagurio in preparing this article.

References

EFFECT OF CORTICOSTEROIDS IN HBsAG-POSITIVE CAH
Biologic Studies
1. Wands JR, Perrotto JL, Alpert E, et al: Cell-mediated immunity in acute and chronic hepatitis. *J Clin Med Invest* 1975; 55:921–929.
2. Sagnelli E, Manzillo G, Maio G, et al: Serum levels of hepatitis B surface and core antigens during immunosuppressive treatment of HBsAg positive chronic active hepatitis. *Lancet* 1980; 2:395–397.
3. Scullard GH, Smith CI, Merigan TC, et al: Effects of immunosuppressive ther-

apy on viral markers in chronic active hepatitis B. *Gastroenterology* 1981; 81:987–999.

Clinical Studies

4. Cook GC, Mulligan R, Sherlock S: Controlled trials of corticosteroid therapy in chronic active hepatitis. *Q J Med* 1971; 40:159–185.

5. Soloway RD, Summerskill WHJ, Baggenstoss AH, et al: Clinical biochemical and histological remission of severe chronic active liver disease: A controlled study of treatment and early prognosis. *Gastroenterology* 1972; 63:820–833.

6. Murray-Lion IM, Stern RB, Williams R: Controlled trial of prednisone and azathioprine in active chronic hepatitis. *Lancet* 1973; 1:735–737.

7. Schalm SW, Summerskill WHJ, Gitnick GL, et al: Contrasting features of severe chronic active liver disease with and without hepatitis Bs antigen. *Gut* 1976; 17:1422–1430.

8. De Groote J, Favery J, Lepoutre L: Long-term follow-up of chronic active hepatitis of moderate severity. *Gut* 1978; 19:510–513.

9. Mayer zum Buschenfelde KH, Creutzfeldt W, Scheurlen, et al: Immunosuppressive therapie der HBs-antigen-positiven und -negativen chronisch-aktiven hepatitis. *Dtsch Med Wochenschr* 1978; 103:887–892.

10. Tsuji T, Naiko K, Tokuyama K, et al: Follow-up ten years after corticosteroid therapy for chronic active hepatitis type B. *Hepatogastroenterology* 1980; 27:85–90.

11. Lam KC, Lai CL, Ng RP, et al: Deleterious effect of prednisolone in HBsAg-positive chronic active hepatitis. *N Engl J Med* 1981; 304:380–386.

12. Smith CI, Andres LL, Scullard GH, et al: Survival in 279 patients with chronic hepatitis B liver diseases, abstracted. *Hepatology* 1981; 1:548.

13. Romeo F, Cannò G, Polosa P: Contraindication of prednisolone treatment in chronic active type B hepatitis of moderate severity. *Ital J Gastroenterol* 1982; 14:220–224.

14. Rizzetto M, Verme G, Recchia S, et al: Chronic HBsAg hepatitis with intrahepatic expression of the delta antigen: An active and progressive disease unresponsive to immunosuppressive treatment. *Ann Intern Med* 1983; 98:437–444.

15. Sagnelli E, Piccinino F, Manzillo G, et al: Effect of immunosuppressive therapy on HBsAg-positive chronic active hepatitis in relation to presence or absence of HBeAg and anti-HBe. *Hepatology* 1983; 3:690–695.

16. Giusti G, Piccinino F, Galanti B, et al: Immunosuppressive therapy in chronic active hepatitis (CAH): A multicentric retrospective study on 867 patients. *Hepatogastroenterology* 1984; 31:24–29.

17. Sagnelli E, Piccinino F, Pasquale G, et al: Delta agent infection: An unfavourable event in HBsAg-positive chronic hepatitis. *Liver* 1984; 4:170–176.

18. Sherlock S, Thomas HC: Treatment of chronic hepatitis due to hepatitis B virus. *Lancet* 1985; 2:1343–1347.

OTHER STUDIES ON HBSAG-POSITIVE CAH

Immunologic Studies

19. Mondelli M, Eddlestone ALWF: Mechanisms of liver cell injury in acute and chronic hepatitis B. *Semin Liver Dis* 1984; 4:47–58.

Clinical Studies

20. Villa E, Theodossi A, Portmann B, et al: Reactivation of hepatitis B virus infection in two patients: Immunofluorescence studies of liver tissue. *Gastroenterology* 1981; 80:1048–1053.

21. Hoofnagle JH, Dusheico GM, Shafer DF, et al: Reactivation of chronic hepatitis B virus infection by cancer chemotherapy. *Ann Intern Med* 1982; 96:447–449.
22. Tolentino P, Iannuzzi C, Giacchino R: Immunosuppressive treatment of chronic HBsAg-positive hepatitis in childhood. *Infection* 1983; 11:255–259.
23. Vajro P, Orso G, D'Antonio A, et al: Inefficacy of immunosuppressive treatment in HBsAg positive, delta-negative, moderate chronic active hepatitis in children. *J Pediatr Gastroenterol Nutr* 1985; 4:26–31.
24. Maggiore G, Marzani D, De Giacome C: L'hepatite chronique a virus HB de l'enfant: Une etude de vingt-neuf observations. *Seminaires Hopital Paris* 1984; 60:1349–1352.

Negative
Gary L. Davis, M.D.

The controversy over corticosteroid treatment of chronic type B (HB$_s$Ag-positive) hepatitis has its roots in the early studies demonstrating the beneficial effects of immunosuppressive therapy in idiopathic (autoimmune; lupoid) CAH. These studies defined the usual course of idiopathic chronic hepatitis and then, based on this knowledge, justified appropriate treatment end points, assessed treatment responses, and proved efficacy. Unfortunately, the results of these successful trials were then widely extrapolated to other unrelated forms of chronic hepatitis without knowledge of the natural histories, appropriate treatment end points, or degree of steroid responsiveness of those diseases. Thus, despite the lack of clinical data to support its use, corticosteroid treatment for chronic type B hepatitis became commonplace and continues to have its supporters.

The purpose of this chapter is to convince the reader that corticosteroids are ineffective and should not be used in the treatment of chronic type B hepatitis. In making this argument, it is first important to review the natural history of chronic type B hepatitis so that reasonable goals of therapy can be formulated based on an understanding of the course of the disease. With these goals in mind, the results of corticosteroid treatment trials in this disease will be reviewed and treatment alternatives will be discussed.

Natural History

Chronic type B hepatitis develops in approximately 10% of individuals acutely infected with the HBV.[1] Chronic infection is divided into two phases defined by whether or not the HBV is present in blood and/or liver. The initial or replicative phase of chronic infection is characterized by the presence of the complete virus, which is detected serologically by HB$_e$Ag or HBV DNA in blood. Patients are usually symptomatic, and variable degrees of hepatic inflammation occur as manifested by abnormal liver tests and chronic hepatitis on liver biopsy. It is during this replicative phase of infection that patients are infectious and the liver disease is most severe and most likely to progress to cirrhosis.[1]

Each year approximately 15% of patients in the replicative phase will progress to the nonreplicative phase of the disease. This event, which is marked by the loss of HB$_e$Ag and development of anti-HB$_e$ is known as seroconversion. Detectable HBV also disappears in most patients, although HB$_s$Ag persists indefinitely, perhaps owing to incorporation of a portion of HBV DNA into the host DNA (integration). Seroconversion is a major landmark in the evolution of chronic type B hepatitis since symptoms resolve, liver tests normalize, hepatic histology reverts toward normal, and infectivity decreases.[1]

Active liver disease persists in a minority of patients following loss of HB$_e$Ag. Reactivation, characterized by the return of HB$_e$Ag and resumption of active hepatitis, occasionally occurs. In general, however, active hepatitis occurring after seroconversion is due to causes other than the HBV.[1]

Chronic type B hepatitis is usually a clinically and biochemically mild disease. In fact, many patients are completely asymptomatic despite the presence of high titers of the virus. Survival in noncirrhotic patients with chronic type B hepatitis exceeds 90% at 5 years. Survival in the 15% to 20% of patients who eventually develop cirrhosis is reduced. In these patients, estimated 2- and 5-year survivals are 70% and 55%, respectively.[2]

Goals of Treatment

It is obvious from the above discussion that the liabilities of chronic type B hepatitis occur during the replicative phase. It is during this time that liver disease progresses and cirrhosis develops. Development of cirrhosis shortens survival. Symptoms occur and infectivity is greatest during the replicative phase. Seroconversion and the resulting loss of virus alleviates these problems. Clearly, the goal of any form of therapy should be to shorten the duration of the replicative phase and rid the host of the virus. The specific goals of treatment in chronic type B hepatitis are given in Table 1. The first four of these are accomplished by shortening the replicative phase of infection. The fifth, prevention of viral DNA integration, is probably important in preventing the late complications of the infection, such as hepatocellular carcinoma. This may be possible by eliminating the

---

TABLE 1.
Specific Goals of Treatment in Patients With Chronic Type B Hepatitis

1. Loss of HB$_e$Ag (seroconversion)
2. Prevention of progressive disease, i.e., development of cirrhosis
3. Decreased infectivity
4. Increased survival
5. Prevention of HBV DNA integration

virus early in the course of chronic infection, but the data are not yet clear. Reduction of serum ALT and aspartate aminotransferase levels usually follows elimination of HBV, but biochemical improvement itself is not a primary goal of therapy since hepatic disease may continue or progress despite improvement of aminotransferase levels.

Experience With Corticosteroid Therapy

Corticosteroid treatment has detrimental effects on the course of acute type B hepatitis. It prolongs prodromal symptoms,[3] decreases early survival,[4] and promotes development of chronic type B hepatitis.[5] These sequelae may occur as the result of steroid inhibition of production of antiviral and immunomodulatory lymphokines, such as interferons, during the acute infection.

As discussed earlier, the rationale for the use of corticosteroids in chronic type B hepatitis was based on early experience with steroids in a different disease, i.e., idiopathic (autoimmune) CAH. As we now know, the natural histories of the two diseases are quite different, and therefore the expectations and results of treatment are not comparable. In addition, the recent observations that corticosteroids increase replication of the HBV (in vitro and in vivo)[6, 7] and inhibit antiviral immunomodulatory mechanisms (e.g., interferon actions) suggest that steroids would not be effective in this disease.[8]

The results of the trials of corticosteroids in chronic type B hepatitis are summarized in Table 2. The patients included in many of the earlier studies are poorly characterized in terms of severity of illness and presence of viral replication. This reflects the lack of knowledge of the natural history of the disease and the unavailability of assays of viral replication. A few reports separated patient groups according to the replicative and non-replicative phases of infection and are perhaps more valid studies.

Early uncontrolled reports demonstrated that corticosteroids were frequently associated with improvement of liver tests and survival approaching 90%.[5, 9-13] These results were considered excellent using the standards derived from studies in patients with idiopathic chronic hepatitis. However, the survival figures are not different from what would be expected without treatment and, considering the severity of the disease and short duration of follow-up in these studies, might even be less than expected. Both Schalm et al.[9] and Tage-Jensen et al.[13] found that survival was especially poor in steroid-treated cirrhotic patients. Noncirrhotic patients did not escape the detrimental effects of treatment either. Follow-up liver biopsies demonstrated histologic progression of disease, with as many as 71% of these steroid-treated patients developing cirrhosis. Finally, steroid treatment appeared to prevent loss of HB$_e$Ag. Although spontaneous termination of the replicative phase (seroconversion) would be expected to occur

TABLE 2.
Clinical Results With Long-term Corticosteroid Administration*

	Source, Yr	No. of Patients	Biochemical Improvement, %	Histologic Progression, %	Raw Survival, %	Frequent Relapses, %	Effect of Steroids
Uncontrolled	Dudley et al.[5] 1972	59	100	65	85	+	Clinical benefit, histologic progression
	Schalm et al.[9] 1976	13	46	...	69	+	Clinical benefit, high mortality
	De Groote et al.,[10] 1978	17	...	71	71	+	Histologic progression
	Meyer zum Buschenfelde,[11] 1978	22	23	82	86	...	Ineffective
	Tolentino et al.,[12] 1983	104	73	...	97	+	Clinical benefit, no seroconversion
	Tage-Jensen et al.,[13] 1985	8	50	...	63	...	Ineffective
	Totals or averages	223	73	69	87	...	...
Untreated controlled	Tsuji et al.,[14] 1980	21/15	67/0	...	86/43	...	Clinical benefit
	Giusti et al.,[15] 1981	59/21	56/0	...	95/96	...	Clinical benefit
	Lam et al.,[16] 1981	25/26	93/88	38/10	72/69	43/22	Ineffective
	EASL,[17] 1984	47/47	...	...	81/96	...	Decreased survival
	Sagnelli et al.,[18] 1983	94/43	39/19	10/20	100/88	52/...	Decreased seroconversion, frequent reactivation
	Vajro et al.,[19] 1985	8/7	39/71	14/0	62/57	+/+	Ineffective
	Total or average	254/159	53/32	16/14	90/82	50/22	...

*Summary data for the above studies were calculated by the author from available data when numbers were not specifically stated in the studies. Data of untreated controlled studies are presented as treated/control. The studies by Tsuji et al.[14] and Giusti et al.[15] were not randomized. EASL indicates European Association for the Study of the Liver.

in about 15% of patients annually, Tolentino et al.[12] found no patients who lost HB$_e$Ag during 2 years of steroid treatment. Davis found a seroconversion rate of only 3% per year.[21] Evidence of reactivation of infection manifested by relapse of disease activity was found in all studies in which it was sought.

Several controlled trials comparing corticosteroids with untreated counterparts have been reported (see Table 2).[14–19] Tsuji and colleagues[14] in a retrospective review found increased survival and diminished disease activity in steroid-treated patients. Giusti et al.,[15] also in a retrospective study, found that steroid-treated patients were more likely to improve biochemically and less likely to deteriorate or develop cirrhosis. Survival was not affected. It is important to point out that these two reports represent the only two controlled studies that suggest a beneficial effect of corticosteroids in this disease. Both studies were retrospective. Neither study was randomized. Four randomized studies comparing corticosteroid treatment with untreated controls have been conducted (see Table 2).[16–19] All four demonstrated that corticosteroids are ineffective and may be detrimental in the treatment of these patients. The first study, by Lam and associates[16] in Hong Kong, concluded that steroids delayed biochemical remission, promoted histologic progression and development of cirrhosis, hastened relapse, and decreased early survival. Unfortunately, this study was flawed in design, execution, and statistical analysis.[20] Despite its shortcomings, it is evident that treated patients were more likely to develop progressive and relapsing disease. The European Association for the Study of the Liver multicenter study was stopped after 4 years because of statistically significant mortality in the steroid-treated group.[17] Sagnelli and colleagues[18] found that prednisone with or without azathioprine did not significantly alter the clinical or biochemical course of chronic type B hepatitis. Vajro et al.[19] demonstrated that steroid treatment had no effect on the course of disease in children.

Table 3 summarizes the few studies that allow analysis of treatment results for patients in the replicative phase (HB$_e$Ag positive) of infection. As already discussed, these are the patients with potentially progressive disease in whom an effective treatment would be desirable. The results of both uncontrolled and controlled studies are similar. The HB$_e$Ag-positive patients treated with steroids were more likely than their untreated counterparts to experience histologic progression of disease and develop cirrhosis. They were far less likely to lose HB$_e$Ag and enter the nonreplicative phase of infection. There was no apparent clinical, biochemical, or survival benefit in the controlled studies of Sagnelli et al.[18] and Vajro et al.[19] Similar observations have been made in HB$_s$Ag-positive patients undergoing renal transplantation who were maintained on a chronic immunosuppressive regimen comprising steroids and azathioprine.[22] These patients had a striking tendency to progression and development of cirrhosis. Patients undergoing transplant who are HBeAg positive rarely seroconvert. In sum-

TABLE 3.
Clinical Results in HB$_e$Ag-Positive Patients With Chronic HB$_s$Ag-Positive Hepatitis*

	Source	No. of Patients	Biochemical Improvement, %	Histologic Progression, %	Developed Cirrhosis, %	Annual Rate HB$_e$Ag Seroconversion, %	Raw Survival, %	Comments
Uncontrolled	Tage-Jensen et al.[13]	4	75	...	...	...	50	Ineffective, bad in cirrhotics
	Davis et al.[21]	15	...	...	80	3.3	73	...
Placebo controlled	Sagnelli et al.[18]	25/12	24/33	20/0	22/22	2/16	100/100	Ineffective
	Vajro et al.[19]	6/4	...	14/0	14/0	16/25	100/100	Ineffective
Total or average	...	50/35	21/33	19/0	33/14	4/19	88/100	...

*Summary data for the above studies were calculated by the author from available data when numbers were not specifically stated in the articles. Placebo-controlled data are presented as treated/control.

mary, corticosteroid treatment is of no benefit in HB_eAg-positive patients and prolongs the replicative phase of the infection, thus increasing the risk of disease progression, development of cirrhosis, and HBV DNA integration while prolonging symptomatic liver disease and the period of infectivity.

The effect of corticosteroid treatment on HB_eAg-negative patients with chronic type B hepatitis is far less clear. In general, these patients would not be expected to have active liver disease since they are usually in the nonreplicative phase of infection. Thus, this atypical group of patients probably represents a mixture of HB_sAg-positive patients with either occult HBV replication or superimposed forms of non-B disease such as delta agent infection, non-A, non-B hepatitis, or idiopathic chronic hepatitis. In no study that identified HB_eAg-negative patients have these other diseases been ruled out. This makes interpretation of results difficult if not impossible. Sagnelli et al.[18] showed an insignificant trend toward increased survival in steroid-treated HB_eAg-negative patients, but treatment frequently induced reactivation with return of HB_eAg and active hepatitis. Reactivation is also common in steroid-treated patients undergoing renal transplant who have anti-HB_e–positive chronic type B hepatitis.[22]

After the first studies citing the potentially detrimental effects of corticosteroid therapy were reported, therapy was discontinued in many patients. A number of investigators observed that some patients lost HB_eAg and developed anti-HB_e following steroid withdrawal (Table 4).[7, 23, 24] However, a subsequent uncontrolled prospective study and two controlled studies of short-term steroid administration and withdrawal failed to confirm the previously observed beneficial effects.[25–27] In retrospect, corticosteroids probably delayed spontaneous seroconversion until the drug was withdrawn. Steroid withdrawal, even after a short course of the drug, may cause exacerbation of disease activity in many patients. In the study reported by Nair et al.,[26] 50% of patients experienced biochemical worsening of their liver disease and 33% developed ascites or variceal hemorrhage with hepatic encephalopathy.

Alternative Treatments

Antiviral agents (adenine arabinoside, adenine arabinoside-monophosphate, acyclovir, interferon) and immunomodulatory agents (interferon, levamisole, transfer factor, immune RNA) have been tested as potential treatments for patients with chronic type B hepatitis. Interferon currently holds the greatest promise as a single agent, with induced seroconversion rates averaging 34%. Early evidence suggests that short courses (3 to 4 months) of interferon in combination with other agents may induce seroconversion in more than 50% of patients.[28]

TABLE 4.
Clinical and Serologic Results of Corticosteroid Withdrawal in HBeAg-Positive Patients With Chronic HBsAg-Positive Hepatitis*

Source, Yr	No. of Patients	HBeAg to Anti-HBe Seroconversion, %	Postwithdrawal Exacerbation, %
Uncontrolled			
Scullard et al.,[7] 1981	3	33	...
Muller et al.,[23] 1981	11	45	...
Hoofnagle and Schafer,[24] 1983	15	47	...
Rakela et al.,[25] 1983	6	0	15
Nair et al.,[26] 1985	11/14	18/0	50
Placebo controlled			
Hoofnagle et al.,[27] 1986	10/5	0/0	20

*Summary data for the above studies were calculated by the author from available data when numbers were not specifically stated in the articles. Placebo-controlled data are presented as treated/control. Studies by Rakela et al.,[25] Nair et al.,[26] and Hoofnagle et al.[27] were prospective.

Summary

The goal of any treatment of chronic type B hepatitis is to eliminate the HBV. Serologically, this translates into loss of HB_eAg and development of anti-HB_e (seroconversion). A loss or significant reduction in infectivity is implied. Coincident with seroconversion is a resolution of disease activity associated with loss of symptoms, normalization of serum liver enzyme tests, reduction of hepatic inflammation, and a decreased chance of progressive disease leading to cirrhosis, hepatocellular failure, or death.

Prolonged administration of corticosteroids has a detrimental effect in patients with chronic type B hepatitis. In HB_eAg-positive patients, steroids prevent seroconversion and thus prolong the replicative phase of disease. The obvious effect is to extend the period of infectivity. The persistence of viral replication also fuels continued hepatic inflammation, resulting in histologic progression and development of cirrhosis, even though liver enzymes often paradoxically improve. Prolongation of the replicative phase may also facilitate integration of HBV DNA into the host genome, although this remains speculative. In HB_eAg-negative patients, corticosteroids induce reactivation of the HBV, thus reintroducing them to the risks and liabilities of the replicative phase of infection described above. In all patients there is a significant and cumulative risk of severe steroid-related side effects.

Use of short courses of corticosteroid administration followed by abrupt withdrawal is to be condemned. Controlled prospective studies have now shown this treatment to be ineffective in causing seroconversion, and the risks of inducing hepatocellular failure are significant.

The clinician is often in the situation of caring for desperately ill patients for whom no treatment exists. In the case of chronic type B hepatitis, these patients are often reflexly treated with steroids. However, since no significant beneficial effects have been proved and the detrimental effects are many, corticosteroid treatment cannot be justified on either a scientific or a humanitarian basis. In conclusion, corticosteroids alone or in combination with azathioprine have no place in the treatment of patients with chronic type B hepatitis.

References

1. Hoofnagle JH, Davis GL, Hanson RG: Chronic hepatitis: Clinical course, in Verme G, Bonino F, Rizzetto M (eds): *Viral Hepatitis and Delta Infection.* New York, Alan R Liss Inc, 1983, pp 41–53.
2. Weissberg JI, Andres LJ, Smith CI, et al: Survival in chronic hepatitis B: An analysis of 379 patients. *Ann Intern Med* 1984; 101:613–616.
3. Johnson BE, Reed JS: Prolongation of the prodrome to acute hepatitis B infection by corticosteroids. *Arch Intern Med* 1983; 143:1810–1811.

4. Greenberg HB, Robinson WS, Knauer CM, et al: Hepatitis B viral markers in severe viral hepatitis: Influence of steroid therapy. *Hepatology* 1981; 1:54–57.
5. Dudley FJ, Scheuer PJ, Sherlock S: Natural history of hepatitis-associated antigen-positive chronic liver disease. *Lancet* 1972; 2:1388–1393.
6. Tur-Kaspa B, Burk RD, Shafritz DA: A glucocorticoid responsive element in the hepatitis B virus genome which enhances viral gene expression. *Hepatology* 1985; 5:1018.
7. Scullard GH, Robinson WS, Merigan TC, et al: The effect of immunosuppressive therapy on viral markers in patients with chronic active hepatitis. *Gastroenterology* 1981; 81:987–991.
8. Berman B, Smith B, Duncan MR: Glucocorticoids inhibit gamma interferon production of HLA-DR antigen expression, abstracted. *Clin Res* 1986; 34:737A.
9. Schalm SW, Summerskill WHJ, Gitnick GL, et al: Contrasting features and responses to treatment of severe chronic active liver disease with and without hepatitis Bs antigen. *Gut* 1976; 17:781–786.
10. De Groote J, Fevery J, Lepoutre L: Long-term follow-up of chronic active hepatitis of moderate severity. *Gut* 1978; 19:510–513.
11. Meyer zum Buschenfelde KH: Immunosuppressive therapie der HBs-antigen-positiven und -negativen chronisch-aktiven hepatitis. *Dtsch Med Wochenschr* 1978; 103:887–892.
12. Tolentino P, Jannuzzi C, Giacchino R: Immunosuppressive treatment of chronic HBsAg-positive hepatitis in childhood. *Infection* 1983; 5:255–259.
13. Tage-Jensen U, Aldershville J, Schlichting P, et al: Immunosuppressive treatment of HBsAg-positive chronic liver disease: Significance of HBeAg. *Hepatology* 1985; 1:47–49.
14. Tsuji T, Naito K, Tokuyama K, et al: Follow-up ten years after corticosteroid therapy for chronic active hepatitis type B. *Hepatogastroenterology* 1980; 27:85–90.
15. Giusti G, Ruggieri G, Galanti B, et al: Treatment of chronic active hepatitis: A retrospective review of 130 patients. *Hepatogastroenterology* 1981; 28:245–249.
16. Lam KC, Lai CL, Ng RP, et al: Deleterious effect of prednisolone in HBsAg-positive chronic active hepatitis. *N Engl J Med* 1981; 304:380–386.
17. European Association for the Study of the Liver: A multicenter randomized clinical trial of low-dose steroid treatment in chronic active HBsAg positive liver disease. *Gastroenterology* 1984; 86:1317.
18. Sagnelli E, Piccinino F, Manzillo G, et al: Effect of immunosuppressive therapy on HBsAg-positive chronic active hepatitis in relation to presence or absence of HBeAg and anti-HBe. *Hepatology* 1983; 3:690–695.
19. Vajro P, Orso G, D'Antonio A, et al: Inefficacy of immunosuppressive treatment in HBsAg-positive, delta-negative, moderate chronic active hepatitis in children. *J Pediatr Gastroenterol Nutr* 1985; 4:26–31.
20. Conn HO, Maddrey WC, Soloway RD: The detrimental effects of adrenocorticosteroid therapy in HBsAg-positive chronic active hepatitis: Fact or artifact. *Hepatology* 1982; 6:885–887.
21. Davis GL, Czaja AJ, Taswell HF, et al: Hepatitis B virus replication in steroid-treated severe HBsAg-positive chronic active hepatitis. *Dig Dis Sci* 1985; 30:97–103.

22. Dusheiko G, Song E, Bowyer S, et al: Natural history of hepatitis B virus infection in renal transplant recipients: A 15 year follow-up. *Hepatology* 1983; 3:330–336.
23. Muller R, Vido I, Schmidt FW: The effect of rapid withdrawal of immunosuppressive therapy in patients with chronic active hepatitis B, in Szmuness W, Alter HJ, Maynard JE (eds): *Viral Hepatitis: 1981 International Symposium.* Philadelphia, Franklin Institute Press, 1981, p 647.
24. Hoofnagle JH, Schafer DF: Management of patients with chronic type B hepatitis, in Cohen S, Soloway RD (eds): *Chronic Active Liver Disease.* New York, Churchill Livingstone, Inc, 1983, pp 81–91.
25. Rakela J, Redeker AG, Weliky B: Effect of short-term prednisone therapy on aminotransferase levels and hepatitis B virus markers in chronic type B hepatitis. *Gastroenterology* 1983; 84:956–960.
26. Nair PV, Tong MJ, Stevenson D, et al: Effects of short-term, high-dose prednisone treatment of patients with HBsAg-positive chronic active hepatitis. *Liver* 1985; 5:8–12.
27. Hoofnagle JH, Davis GL, Pappas SC, et al: A short course of prednisolone in chronic type B hepatitis: Report of a randomized, double-blind, placebo-controlled trial. *Ann Intern Med* 1986; 104:12–17.
28. Davis GL, Hoofnagle JH: Interferon in viral hepatitis: Role in pathogenesis and treatment. *Hepatology,* in press.

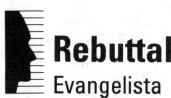

Rebuttal: Affirmative
Evangelista Sagnelli, M.D.

I enjoyed reading Dr. Davis' article, in which he endeavored to convince the reader that corticosteroids are ineffective and should not be used in the treatment of chronic type B hepatitis, but I found that he wandered slightly from the subject. The question is "should some patients with chronic *active* hepatitis B be treated with corticosteroids?" Well, although Dr. Davis did not state outright that no patient with CAH should be treated with corticosteroids, his message seems to be that, in general, this treatment is ineffective in chronic hepatitis B.

Dr. Davis began his statement by outlining the natural history of chronic hepatitis B, which is still a rather obscure matter. Not even the data published by Hoofnagle et al.[1] in 1983, quoted several times by Dr. Davis, have clarified the natural history of chronic hepatitis B, largely because the course of the disease was evaluated only on the bases of clinical and biochemical data. Consequently, Dr. Davis' statement that "It is during this replicative phase of infection that . . . the liver disease is most severe and most likely to progress to cirrhosis" is not supported by unquestionable evidence.

In reality, Dr. Davis deals with the natural history of HBV infection rather than with that of CAH and, with the exception of seroconversion to anti-HB$_e$, fails to mention any other immunologic phenomena probably involved in the pathogenesis of this disease. Consequently, the clinical course of the different types of HB$_s$Ag-positive chronic hepatitis (namely, chronic persistent hepatitis [CPH], chronic lobular hepatitis [CLH], and CAH) were rarely evaluated separately, and progression to cirrhosis was connected only with the failure to seroconvert to anti-HB$_e$. Unfortunately, things are more complex, as the reader may realize by reading recent reviews by Mondelli and Eddleston[2] and by Dienstag[3] on immunologic mechanisms in chronic viral hepatitis.

There is a sentence in Dr. Davis' article that really surprised me. He describes patients with HB$_e$Ag-negative CAH as an atypical group of patients representing "a mixture of HB$_s$Ag-positive patients with either occult HBV replication or superimposed forms of non-B disease such as delta agent infection, non-A, non-B hepatitis, or idiopathic chronic hepatitis." However, 35% of our patients with HB$_s$Ag-positive CAH lacked serum HB$_e$Ag, HBV DNA, and anti-HD. This prevalence is even higher in most geographic areas where HDV infection is infrequent. It is hard to believe that in 35% or more of patients with HB$_s$Ag-positive CAH the disease is due to nonidentifiable agents. We have no evidence to support this.

Dr. Davis attentively reviewed the available data on corticosteroid therapy of HB$_s$Ag-positive CAH. We both agree that patients with HBV replication should not be treated with these drugs, whereas we have different opinions about HBV DNA–negative patients. Whether liver disease progresses and cirrhosis develops during HBV replication or later, and whether or not one wishes to hypothesize that nonidentifiable agents are responsible for the active phase of the disease, the fact remains that these patients still need to be treated. Naturally, antiviral therapy is not indicated in the absence of viral replication. At this point, should HBV DNA–negative patients with CAH be treated with corticosteroids? Dr. Davis' chapter seems to suggest they should not. In my opinion this is correct when patients have established cirrhosis (they may worsen under immunosuppressive therapy) and when they show moderately active CAH. I do believe that patients with severe and sometimes symptomatic CAH should be considered for corticosteroid treatment, especially in view of the fact that no other treatment has been shown effective. In my experience, about 50% of them have shown clinical, biochemical, and histologic improvement when treated with a combination of 20 mg of prednisolone daily and of 50 mg of azathioprine daily.

In response to Dr. Davis' statement that relapses after discontinuation of treatment are an important drawback of corticosteroid therapy, I maintain that relapses may be harmful in patients with cirrhosis, who may develop variceal hemorrhage with hepatic encephalopathy or ascites, whereas in CAH without cirrhosis the exacerbation of the disease is frequently moderate and followed by remission, and only in a few cases does it lead to severe or fatal hepatitis. However, patients may repeatedly discontinue and resume taking corticosteroids by themselves and in so doing run the risk of several relapses. In my experience this is harmful even to patients with CAH without cirrhosis. On the whole, relapses should be avoided or at least limited by a gradual breaking off of immunosuppressive therapy.

In conclusion, the chapter by Dr. Davis does not convince me that no patient with HB$_s$Ag-positive CAH should be treated with corticosteroids. However, I must say that these drugs do not solve the problem of treatment of HB$_s$Ag-positive CAH, and that new drugs (not only antiviral) should be evaluated. Until new effective treatment becomes available, corticosteroids given in association with azathioprine may be considered for treating patients with CAH, whether symptomatic or asymptomatic, with the following characteristics: severe histologic lesions, no established cirrhosis, and no serum markers of HBV replication.

References

1. Hoofnagle JH, Davis GL, Hanson RG: Chronic hepatitis: Clinical course, in Verme G, Bonino F, Rizzetto M (eds): *Viral Hepatitis and Delta Infection*. New York, Alan R Liss Inc, 1983, pp 41–53.

2. Mondelli M, Eddleston ALWF: Mechanisms of liver cell injury in acute and chronic hepatitis B. *Semin Liver Dis* 1984; 4:47–58.
3. Dienstag JL: Immunologic mechanisms in chronic viral hepatitis, in Vyas GN, Dienstag JL, Hoofnagle JH (eds): *Viral Hepatitis and Liver Disease.* New York, Grune & Stratton, 1984, pp 135–166.

Rebuttal: Negative
Gary L. Davis, M.D.

The major concerns about the use of corticosteroids in the treatment of chronic type B hepatitis are the perpetuation and possible enhancement of HBV replication, potential exacerbations of hepatic inflammation, drug-induced side effects, and decreased survival. It is difficult to argue with the fact that these concerns far outweigh the slight chance of any potential benefit derived from steroid treatment in patients with chronic type B hepatitis. In fact, much of the substance of the affirmative statement agrees with my view that corticosteroids are ineffective and potentially harmful in the treatment of these patients. Dr. Sagnelli concurs that corticosteroid treatment should not be offered to patients who are HB_eAg positive, have cirrhosis, or have only mild disease. The only area of disagreement is whether or not immunosuppressive treatment is of benefit in anti-HB_e–positive patients.

As discussed earlier, the majority of anti-HB_e–positive patients do not have active liver disease or evidence of HBV replication. Matsuyama et al.[1] found that 18% of anti-HB_e–positive patients had HBV DNA detected in serum. I have found this to occur much less frequently and usually only transiently within the first few months after seroconversion. Serum aminotransferase levels are usually not greatly elevated in these patients, and nearly half will have cirrhosis. Such patients are more likely to reactivate with reversion to HB_eAg positivity, especially if they are immunosuppressed.[2] There are several reasons why anti-HB_e–positive patients with persistent HBV replication should not be treated. First, disease is mild in most of these patients. Second, these patients behave like HB_eAg-positive patients (active liver disease, HBV DNA positive), and steroids would be expected to prolong and possibly worsen their disease. Third, steroids frequently will cause reactivation. And finally, since we know that steroids dramatically reduce survival in cirrhotic patients with chronic type B hepatitis, the predictable mortality in these particular anti-HB_e–positive patients would be significant.

Most anti-HB_e–positive patients do not have persistent HBV replication, however. When hepatic inflammatory activity persists in these patients, other causes of active liver disease such as non-A, non-B hepatitis, idiopathic (autoimmune) hepatitis, alcoholic liver disease, or drug reaction should be considered. Delta agent is another cause of active disease in these patients and is especially common in Italy. Approximately 70% of the patients in Dr. Sagnelli's studies are delta agent positive. This fact may explain some of the findings of his studies in anti-HB_e–positive patients.[3] The number of patients who deteriorated with or without therapy (nearly 50%) is not consistent with chronic type B hepatitis but is typical of delta agent superinfection.[4] The similarity of treatment responses between steroid-treated and untreated patients is compatible with the findings of others that steroids are not effective in delta agent infection.[5] The finding of significantly less deterioration in Sagnelli's prednisone/azathioprine group may be related to a smaller number of delta agent–infected patients in that treatment group. These questions are not answered in his article. The only other study to address steroid treatment of anti-HB$_e$–positive patients failed to find any beneficial effect.[6] Only four such patients were studied, but one died and three had reversion to HB$_e$Ag with reactivation of their liver disease. These episodes of steroid-induced reactivation are especially dangerous in patients with chronic type B hepatitis. Reactivation leads to severe exacerbation of hepatic inflammation and a likelihood of progressive liver disease, e.g., development of cirrhosis. In cirrhotic patients, reactivation may be fatal.

In summary, there is no good evidence from available studies that corticosteroids are of benefit in any patient with chronic type B hepatitis. At best, they are ineffective. At worst, they may result in prolongation and progression of active disease, reactivation of inactive disease, or death.

References

1. Matsuyama Y, Omata M, Yokosuka O, et al: Discordance of hepatitis B e antigen/antibody and hepatitis B virus deoxyribonucleic acid in serum. Analysis of 1063 specimens. *Gastroenterology* 1985; 89:1104–1108.
2. Dusheiko G, Song E, Bowyer S, et al: Natural history of hepatitis B virus infection in renal transplant recipients: A 15 year follow-up. *Hepatology* 1983; 3:330–336.
3. Sagnelli E, Piccinino F, Manzillo G, et al: Effect of immunosuppressive therapy on HBsAg-positive chronic active hepatitis in relation to presence or absence of HBeAg and anti-HBe. The delta. *Hepatology* 1983; 3:690–695.
4. Rizzetto M: *Hepatology* 1983; 3:729–737.
5. Rizzetto M, Verme G, Recchia S, et al: Chronic hepatitis in carriers of hepatitis B surface antigen, with intrahepatic expression of the delta antigen: An active and progressive disease unresponsive to immunosuppressive treatment. *Ann Intern Med* 1983; 98:437–441.
6. Tage-Jensen U, Aldershville J, Schlichting P, et al: Immunosuppressive treatment of HBsAg-positive chronic liver disease: Significance of HBeAg. *Hepatology* 1985; 1:47–49.

Editor's Comments
Gary Gitnick, M.D.

Both Dr. Sagnelli and Dr. Davis have provided cogent arguments. Both interpret the same literature in differing ways. Whereas Dr. Davis eloquently quotes the literature and bases his argument on this, Dr. Sagnelli clearly points out flaws in the existing literature, noting deficiencies where they exist. He tends to substantiate his arguments utilizing his own extensive personal experience, as well as several retrospective or inadequately controlled studies. In spite of the problems in the literature, the two debators have come to opposing conclusions.

Dr. Davis makes the important distinction that patients with CAH may be segregated into those whose disease is in the replicative phase or a phase in which live virus exists, and those who are in the integrated phase in which presumably viral DNA has become integrated into hepatocellular DNA and in which live virus no longer is present. He points out that it is in the replicative phase that the disease progresses and cirrhosis develops. One might question this conclusion, although most would agree that in the replicative phase cellular destruction might occur. There actually is no evidence that the hepatitis virus is cytolytic. In fact, the available data suggest that immune mediation subsequent to infection and replication probably leads to progressive cellular destruction. One might also argue whether the replicative phase is actually associated with the development of cirrhosis, although cirrhosis does indeed occur subsequent to the destructive, inflammatory, and reparative phases. Data establishing that cirrhosis develops in the replicative and not in the integrative phase are lacking. Nevertheless, his conclusion that "clearly the goal of any form of therapy should be to shorten the duration of the replicative phase and rid the host of the virus" is admirable. He follows this with another important point that, although the aminotransferase levels usually are reduced after elimination of HBV infection, it is not a primary goal of therapy since liver disease may progress in spite of improvement in aminotransferase levels. Too often patients and physicians rely on the aminotransferase levels as indicators of the status of chronic liver disease, a reliance that is not established by the available data. He quotes the literature extensively to support his contention that corticosteroid therapy is detrimental in the course of chronic hepatitis B. However, he utilizes references, many of which do not differentiate the results of corticosteroid treatment in patients in the replicative phase as compared with those in the integrated phase.

Dr. Sagnelli would stress that there is a paucity of control data evaluating corticosteroid treatment among patients with chronic hepatitis B who are in the integrative phase. Indeed, most studies have utilized patients who have evidence of replication, such as HB_e antigen or DNA polymerase, and have extrapolated these data to patients who lack these indexes of active viral infection. Nevertheless, Dr. Davis makes strong and convincing arguments. This editor would agree that the available data overwhelmingly oppose the use of corticosteroids in patients in the replicative phase of disease, that is, those who are HB_eAg positive or who carry DNA polymerase. Furthermore, the presence of cirrhosis also indicates little likelihood that corticosteroids can be of help.

However, Dr. Davis has not convinced me that the patient in the integrated phase cannot benefit from corticosteroids. Admittedly, properly designed studies evaluating such patients are lacking, and it is in this group that Dr. Sagnelli makes the strongest arguments. One area of agreement between both debators is that patients with established cirrhosis should not be treated with corticosteroids. I join in this conclusion. Dr. Sagnelli concedes that patients with mild CAH should be left untreated until more effective drugs become available. This leaves for consideration noncirrhotic patients with severe CAH who lack evidence of active viral replication (HB_eAg or DNA polymerase). Indeed, Dr. Sagnelli goes one step further and states that immunosuppressive therapy should be considered only for the anti-HB_e-positive patient without cirrhosis but with severe disease. Nevertheless, he goes on to cite anecdotal evidence of patients who lack these criteria who also improved. Dr. Davis retorts by pointing out that in one study 18% of anti-HB_e–positive patients had HBV DNA detected in serum, although in his experience this occurs less frequently. Thus, the candidates for treatment may be narrowed even further to those who have severe disease, lack cirrhosis, have anti-HB_e, but lack HB_eAg, DNA polymerase, and HBV DNA. Dr. Davis then also effectively argues that those who have active delta infection have been shown not to respond to immunosuppressive treatment.

Thus, I could conclude from the arguments presented by both authors that most patients with CAH should not be treated with immunosuppressive treatment. There is one small group for whom controversy continues regarding the indications for treatment. These are patients with severe CAH, who lack evidence of cirrhosis, who carry anti-HB_e, but who lack markers of active viral replication, such as HB_eAg, DNA polymerase, HBV DNA, and HDV infection. In the absence of a well-designed, prospective, controlled trial, looking at this very select group of patients the reader is left without a database to guide him or her with regard to treating these selected patients. My approach in this small group of patients has been to provide them with a trial of treatment for 6 months. If they improve, I continue the treatment for a full year, and if they fail to improve or if they deteriorate, I stop the treatment. I do not know whether this is right or wrong, and until a proper study is done, none of us will know.

Digitalis Should Be Used to Treat Patients With Congestive Heart Failure

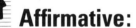

Chapter Editor: Nicholas J. Fortuin, M.D.

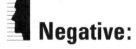

Affirmative: Barry H. Greenberg, M.D.
Professor of Medicine, Director, Coronary
Care Unit, Oregon Health Sciences
University, Portland, Oregon

Negative: Arthur Selzer, M.D.
Clinical Professor of Medicine, University of
California at San Francisco; Clinical
Professor Emeritus, Stanford University
School of Medicine, Stanford, California

Debates in Medicine 1:118–137, 1988
©1988, Year Book Medical Publishers, Inc.
0887-218X/88/01-118-137-$04.00

Affirmative
Barry H. Greenberg, M.D.

Digitalis has been used to treat patients with congestive heart failure (CHF) for over 200 years. During this time, a considerable body of information describing the physiologic effects of digitalis has accumulated in the medical literature and the results of numerous clinical trials have been reported. Despite this abundance of information, there is still no consensus regarding the value of digitalis in the treatment of CHF. Much of the controversy is due to the contradictory results of the physiologic studies that demonstrate clear-cut evidence of improved cardiac performance and some of the clinical trials that fail to show clinical efficacy. In view of the relatively high incidence of digitalis toxicity that was reported during the early 1970s and the recent development of potent diuretics, vasodilators, and other inotropic agents, some authorities now recommend that prescription of digitalis be limited to patients who have a rapid ventricular response to atrial fibrillation. Such a course would, in my opinion, deprive us of an agent that, when used judiciously, is of considerable value in the treatment of CHF. I will review some of the physiologic actions and clinical effects of digitalis so that a rational approach to its use can be developed.

Both animal and human studies show that digitalis increases myocardial contractility in both the normal and the failing heart. In fact, the drug appears to have relatively greater positive inotropic effects when it is given in the setting of depressed myocardial function. However, there are important limitations relevant to its use in patients with CHF. Digitalis does not improve contractility in necrotic myocardium or in scar tisssue, and its cardiotonic effects on severely ischemic myocardium are limited. In addition, the efficacy of digitalis appears to be diminished when myocardium is already being intensely stimulated by catecholamines, as occurs during the course of an acute myocardial infarction (MI). These factors help explain why digitalization of the patient with an acute MI has somewhat variable effects on cardiac performance. Digitalis is also unlikely to be of much value when CHF develops in the presence of normal left ventricular systolic pump function. This situation may occur in patients with mitral stenosis, hypertrophic cardiomyopathy, restrictive cardiomyopathy, pericardial disease, and other conditions where ventricular filling or diastolic function are impaired. Finally, it is worth mentioning that digitalis is a relatively weak inotropic agent compared with isoproterenol or some of the newer agents, such as amrinone or milrinone. However, this may be in the drug's favor since it is probably not advisable to apply too much inotropic stimulation to the failing heart for fear that the "flogging" effect will hasten myocardial deterioration and increase the risk of fatal ventricular arrhythmias. There is some information that the more potent inotropic agents may have such deleterious effects.

119

Although the primary action of digitalis is to improve myocardial contractility, there are other properties of the drug that will influence its effect on cardiac performance in patients with CHF. Digitalis can lead to increased tone in arteries and veins both by a direct effect on vascular smooth muscle and indirectly through the sympathetic nervous system. Enhanced vasomotor tone can have adverse effects on cardiac performance. Constriction of arterial resistance vessels increases the impedance to left ventricular emptying. In patients with left ventricular dysfunction, this may result in a fall in both stroke volume and cardiac output. Constriction of venous capacitance vessels pushes blood that has been pooled in the periphery back to the heart. This effect will tend to increase ventricular filling pressures.

Fortunately, the effects of digitalis on vasomotor tone are strongly influenced by the clinical setting. In patients with CHF, considerable peripheral vasoconstriction is often already present as the body attempts to maintain an adequate arterial perfusion pressure in the face of a reduced cardiac output. The sympathetic nervous system, renin-angiotensin system, and other neurohumoral pathways play key roles in this response. By improving myocardial function and increasing cardiac output, digitalis leads to a withdrawal of vasoconstrictor forces. The net effect in most cases is a reduction rather than an increase in peripheral vasomotor tone. In addition, the vasoconstrictor effects of digitalis are strongly influenced by the rapidity with which the drug is given. When administered as a bolus, substantial increases in systemic vascular resistance as well as end-organ ischemia have been reported. However, when the drug is given in a more leisurely fashion (either by slow infusion or by the oral route), the vasoconstrictor effects are considerably less pronounced.

Finally, digitalis also has an important effect on impulse conduction through the atrioventricular (AV) node. It acts both directly on nodal tissue and indirectly through the parasympathetic nervous system to slow conduction velocity and increase AV nodal refractoriness. These properties make digitalis an effective agent in slowing the ventricular response to atrial fibrillation. About 20% of patients with CHF are in atrial fibrillation, and in most of these patients it is desirable to slow the ventricular response. The disadvantages of a rapid ventricular response are that (1) myocardial oxygen consumption (MVO_2) is increased, (2) stroke volume is diminished and atrial pressures are increased due to the reduction in diastolic filling period, and (3) the ability to respond appropriately to conditions that increase total body oxygen consumption (e.g., exercise) is impaired. In general, a reasonable goal of therapy is to reduce the ventricular response to no greater than 80 or 90 beats per minute at rest and limit the increase that occurs with mild exercise (such as walking on a level or up a flight of stairs) to less than 110 to 120 beats per minute. Other drugs that are capable of slowing conduction through the AV node, such as the β-blockers or verapamil, have important negative inotropic effects, and their administration to patients with CHF may lead to considerable worsening of their condition. Consequently, digitalis is the drug of choice for controlling the ventricular response to atrial fibrillation in patients with CHF.

Despite all of these considerations, clear-cut evidence that digitalis therapy leads to the clinical improvement of patients with CHF has not been consistently available. This is largely due to the fact that virtually all studies that have evaluated the efficacy of digitalis in CHF have had serious design flaws. Insufficient sample size, lack of adequate randomization and blinding, and vague definition of end points make interpretation of many of the trials problematic. In particular, inclusion of patients with normal left ventricular ejection fraction, poorly documented evidence of CHF, hypertrophic or restrictive cardiomyopathy, or pericardial disease have seriously biased many of these studies against showing a positive result. However, when administered to an appropriate group of patients, digitalis can be of considerable value. In a study by Arnold and coworkers from the University of California in San Francisco, the effects of digoxin on cardiac performance were assessed in a group of nine patients who had a well-documented history of CHF and evidence of left ventricular dysfunction. All were in sinus rhythm. Patients were studied at rest and during bicycle exercise using a right-sided heart catheter to measure pressures and flow. Since all patients had been receiving digoxin for their CHF, the initial measurements for the study were obtained while patients were receiving the drug. These measurements were then repeated both after the drug had been withdrawn for a period of several weeks and following acute readministration of digoxin therapy. Clinical deterioration in response to digoxin withdrawal was noted in five (56%) of the nine patients. Rehospitalization for worsening CHF was required in four patients within a month. As assessed by hemodynamic evaluation, cardiac performance deteriorated without the drug in all nine patients. At rest, mean pulmonary artery wedge pressure increased from 21 ± 8 mm Hg at baseline to 29 ± 10 mm Hg and cardiac index had decreased from 2.4 ± 0.7 to 2.1 ± 0.6 L/min/sq m. Ejection fraction had fallen from 0.41 ± 0.14 to 0.30 ± 0.14, and creatinine clearance was reduced from 78 ± 15 to 55 ± 9 ml/min. Cardiac performance during exercise also deteriorated when digoxin was withdrawn. Readministration of drug brought both rest and exercise cardiac performance back to baseline levels. Another convincing study was reported by Lee and coworkers from the Massachusetts General Hospital. They used a randomized, double-blinded, crossover study to compare the effects of digitalis with those produced by a placebo on the severity of CHF in 25 patients who were in normal sinus rhythm. A clinicoradiographic scoring system that correlated closely with measurement of pulmonary artery wedge pressure was used to assess the severity of CHF during the study. In this trial, 14 patients (56%) improved their heart failure score while receiving digitalis. The group of 11 nonresponders tended to give a history of episodic rather than persistent heart failure. Of interest was the fact that six of them had a normal resting ventricular ejection fraction and three of the remaining five patients were asymptomatic during the placebo phase of the trial. This observation highlights the problems inherent in establishing the efficacy of a drug if it is tested in a population that is unlikely to benefit from it. In this study, the reproducibility of the response to digitalis was assessed in six patients, five of whom had responded favorably during the initial comparison of digitalis with placebo. On repeated evaluation, all five of the responders again demonstrated improvement in their CHF when the drug was readministered. For the entire group, the most important predictor of a positive response to digitalis in this study was the presence of an S_3, which was detected in all 14 patients who responded favorably but only in one of the 11 nonresponders.

Since coronary artery disease is an important cause of CHF in the United States and other developed nations, a clinically relevant question is how digitalis affects $M\dot{V}O_2$. Interventions that increase $M\dot{V}O_2$ are undesirable since they would increase the likelihood of myocardial ischemia. The $M\dot{V}O_2$ depends on three factors: (1) intramyocardial tension or wall stress, (2) heart rate, and (3) myocardial contractility. The positive inotropic effects of digitalis tend to increase $M\dot{V}O_2$, and in the absence of heart failure this is what occurs. However, most patients with CHF have cardiomegaly, a factor that favors increased wall stress. By decreasing heart size, digitalis administration tends to reduce wall stress and $M\dot{V}O_2$. In addition, heart rate often falls following digitalization since an improvement in cardiac function usually leads to a withdrawal of sympathetic stimulation. Overall, in patients with CHF these two beneficial effects tend to balance the effect of increased contractility, and the net result is that $M\dot{V}O_2$ is either unchanged or slightly diminished with digitalis.

Recently, retrospective analysis of factors related to survival in several large groups of patients discharged from the hospital following MI have suggested that digitalis therapy appears to have an adverse effect on survival that is independent of its association with other factors such as CHF. Moss and coworkers reported that even after adjustment for relevant nondigitalis risk factor variables such as CHF and complex ventricular arrhythmias, a 30% increase in predicted mortality was seen after 4 months in MI survivors who were taking digitalis. Although statistical methods can adjust for the presence of important confounding variables that affect survival, subtle nuances in a patient's condition that were detected by the primary physician could have led to the prescription of digitalis to a higher-risk population. Such differences in the group that was given digitalis could easily be overlooked when a large population is evaluated retrospectively. In addition, other reports, such as those originating from the Coronary Artery Surgery Study and the Multicenter Investigation of Limitation of Infarct Size, did not support the finding that digitalis administration was an independent risk factor for mortality. Thus, review of the currently available literature fails to demonstrate a consensus in the findings regarding the risk of digitalis in survivors of MI. The only way to address this question adequately is by means of a well-designed clinical trial in which digitalis is randomly prescribed to patients who are then followed up in a prospective fashion.

One of the main concerns about the use of digitalis in CHF is that the drug appears to have a low toxic-therapeutic ratio. Furthermore, toxic manifestations of digitalis can be severe and life-threatening. In a report that appeared in the early 1970s, investigators at the Massachusetts General Hospital found that 23% of hospitalized patients who were receiving digitalis fulfilled definite criteria for digitalis toxicity whereas an additional 6% were possibly toxic. Reports such as this one have alerted practicing clinicians to the magnitude of the problem of digitalis toxicity. This information as well as the widespread availability of laboratory testing to measure serum drug levels has resulted in considerable reduction in the incidence of digitalis toxic reaction today. Often the manifestations of toxicity can be quite subtle. A packaging error that led to an excessive dose of digitalis being given to a large group of patients in the Netherlands allowed investigators to determine the frequency with which noncardiac side effects occurred in patients given toxic doses of the drug. Of note was the high frequency of fatigue and profound muscle weakness, gastrointestinal symptoms, and neuroaffective disorders.

In summary, digitalis is a useful drug for the treatment of CHF. The patients who are most likely to benefit are those with atrial fibrillation since the effects of digitalis on the myocardium and AV nodal tissue combine to improve cardiac function. Digitalis can also benefit patients with CHF who are in normal sinus rhythm provided that it is given in the appropriate setting. When CHF develops as a result of conditions such as mitral stenosis (when the patient is in normal sinus rhythm), pericardial disease, hypertrophic cardiomyopathy, or intermittent left ventricular dysfunction due to myocardial ischemia, digitalis is unlikely to be of much help. Patients with large MIs who develop heart failure acutely will probably also not benefit greatly by digitalis administration. In these groups of patients, other forms of therapy are both more effective and can be administered with less risk than digitalis. Careful consideration of the indications for digitalis use, which include the presence of symptomatic CHF due to left ventricular dysfunction (as manifested by depressed left ventricular ejection fraction) and possibly the presence of a third heart sound, will likely lead to evidence of greater efficacy in clinical practice. The serious toxic potential of digitalis emphasizes the need to evaluate patients carefully so that the drug is prescribed only to patients who both require and will benefit from inotropic support. As already noted, when used judiciously serum digoxin levels are helpful in preventing toxicity and they can also be used to ensure that patients are receiving adequate amounts of drug.

Although digitalis clearly has a place in the treatment of patients with CHF, the therapeutic options that are available for the treatment of this syndrome have expanded considerably over the past two decades. There are now more potent diuretics, clinically effective vasodilator drugs, and even more powerful inotropic agents that can be used to treat patients with CHF. However, evidence demonstrating that these agents are either safer or more effective than digitalis in the treatment of CHF is lacking. In the absence of definitive comparison studies, it would be a great mistake to withhold digitalis from patients who are likely to improve when it is administered.

Bibliography

1. Antman EM, Smith TW: Digitalis toxicity. Mod Concepts Cardiovasc Dis 1986; 55:26–30.
2. Arnold SB, Byrd RC, Meister W, et al: Long-term digitalis therapy improves left ventricular function in heart failure. N Engl J Med 1980; 303:1443.
3. Beller GA, Smith TW, Abelmann W, et al: Digitalis intoxication: A prospective clinical study with serum level correlations. N Engl J Med 1971; 284:989–997.
4. Braunwald E: Effects of digitalis on the normal and the failing heart. J Am Coll Cardiol 1985; 5:51A–59A.
5. DeMots H, Rahimtoola SH, McAnulty JH, et al: Effects of ouabain on coronary and systemic vascular resistance and myocardial oxygen consumption in patients without heart failure. Am J Cardiol 1978; 41:88–93.
6. Goldstein RA, Passamani ER, Roberts R: A comparison of digoxin and dobutamine in patients with acute infarction and cardiac failure. N Engl J Med 1980; 303:846–850.
7. Lee DC, Johnson RA, Bingham JB, et al: Heart failure in outpatients: A new randomized trial of digoxin versus placebo. N Engl J Med 1982; 306:699–705.
8. Lely AH, Van Enter CHJ: Non-cardiac symptoms of digitalis intoxication. Am Heart J 1972; 83:149–152.
9. Longhurst JC, Ross J Jr: Extracardiac and coronary vascular effects of digitalis. J Am Coll Cardiol 1985; 5:99A–105.
10. Madsen EB, Gilpin E, Henning H, et al: Prognostic importance of digitalis after acute myocardial infarction. J Am Coll Cardiol 1984; 3:681–689.
11. Mason DT, Braunwald E: Studies on digitalis: X. Effects of ouabain on forearm vascular resistance and venous tone in normal subjects and in patients in heart failure. J Clin Invest 1964; 43:532–543.
12. Massie B, Bourassa M, DiBianco R, et al: Long-term oral administration of amrinone for congestive heart failure: Lack of efficacy in a multicenter controlled trial. Circulation 1985; 71:963–971.
13. Moss AJ, Davis HT, Conard DL, et al: Digitalis-associated cardiac mortality after myocardial infarction. Circulation 1981; 64:1150–1156.
14. Muller JE, Turi ZG, Stone PH, et al: Digoxin therapy and mortality after myocardial infarction. N Engl J Med 1986; 314:265–271.
15. Mulrow CD, Feussner JR, Velez R: Reevaluation of digitalis efficacy. Ann Intern Med 1984; 101:113–117.
16. O'Rourke RA, Henning H, Theroux P, et al: Favorable effects of orally admin-

istered digoxin on left heart size and ventricular wall motion in patients with previous myocardial infarction. *Am J Cardiol* 1976; 37:708–715.

17. Packer M, Medina N, Yushak M: Hemodynamic and clinical limitations of long-term inotropic therapy with amrinone in patients with severe chronic heart failure. *Circulation* 1984; 70:1039–1047.

18. Raabe DS: Combined therapy with digoxin and nitroprusside in heart failure complicating acute myocardial infarction. *Am J Cardiol* 1979; 43:990–994.

Negative
Arthur Selzer, M.D.

Digitalis exerts several pharmacologic actions on the cardiovascular system. However, from the standpoint of therapy, two effects account for its clinical usefulness: its dromotropic action, slowing conduction across the AV node, and its inotropic action, strengthening the force of cardiac contraction. Both actions play a role in treatment of CHF: dromotropic action slows the rapid ventricular rate in atrial fibrillation, which frequently causes or aggravates heart failure; inotropic action may improve the circulatory dynamics, reducing the consequences of heart failure.

Controversy pertaining to the use of digitalis involves the role played by digitalis in management of cardiac failure in patients who are in sinus rhythm. The point at issue is whether the benefits of digitalis are sufficiently important to balance the generally recognized risks involved in digitalis administration. A corollary to this point is the question whether comparable improvement may be attained by agents associated with lesser risk. Thus, the discussion of the use of digitalis in cardiac failure involves a review of the relationship between the risks and benefits of digitalis.

Risk of Digitalis

That digitalis is one of the most toxic drugs used in cardiac patients is beyond controversy. A number of studies have demonstrated that digitalis intoxication is a common reason for hospitalizing patients with cardiac disease and constitutes an important cause of death. Many properties of digitalis make the possibility of development of digitalis intoxication a real one despite its most cautious use.

Digitalis is a slow-acting drug with a very long half-life (36 hours to 7 days). The universally used digitalis glycoside, digoxin, has a half-life of about 36 hours. Long half-life has both advantages and disadvantages. On the positive side, digitalis needs to be administered only once a day, which facilitates patient compliance; furthermore, omission of one or two doses does not affect its continuous effect on the circulation. On the negative side, slow-acting drugs require large loading doses to initiate treatment; long lag time makes such drugs poorly suitable for treatment of emergencies; and finally, toxic reaction may develop slowly and inconspicuously but persists for a long time when discovered.

Digitalis is a drug with a narrow therapeutic range, i.e., the dose needed to attain the desired effect is close to the toxic dose. The dosage of digitalis necessary to obtain therapeutic effect shows wide individual variation, which is related to variable absorption of the drug (particularly digoxin), to individual sensitivity to the drug, and to a variety of extraneous factors that exert synergistic or antagonistic actions with the drug. It should be emphasized that only the dromotropic action of digitalis can be clinically monitored by observing the ventricular rate in atrial fibrillation, thereby subject to individual adjustment of dosage. The inotropic effect is very difficult, often impossible to judge, particularly since patients in cardiac failure usually require intervention that includes other agents in addition to digitalis. As a consequence, digitalis in sinus rhythm has to be administered blindly, using set dosage schedules without knowledge of whether a given dose schedule is inadequate, correct, or excessive.

The sensitivity of the myocardium to digitalis is subject to change in response to a variety of noncardiac factors. Among those are electrolyte imbalance, particularly hypopotassemia, impaired renal function, hypoxia, old age, and drug interaction (e.g., quinidine). Furthermore, the state of the myocardium itself may determine sensitivity to this drug; impaired myocardial function or myocardial ischemia renders the heart more sensitive to digitalis, so that ordinary doses could produce digitalis toxic reaction.

The development of digitalis toxic reaction occurs by different routes: a mismatch between the dose administered and the sensitivity of the patient may induce toxic reaction initially; gradual development of toxic reaction may occur with a maintenance dose excessive for a given patient. The most difficult to detect, however, is digitalis toxic reaction developing in patients who appear to do well on a given maintenance dosage schedule but in whom an extraneous factor alters sensitivity to digitalis, e.g., hypopotassemia due to vomiting, hypoxia due to bronchitis in a patient with chronic pulmonary disease, or the development of myocardial ischemia or MI.

Manifestations of digitalis toxic reaction include many clinical signs and symptoms that merge with those of CHF and may be difficult to recognize. Both cardiac and extracardiac toxic reaction occurs. Cardiac toxic reaction is more dangerous: it includes a variety of arrhythmias up to and including fatal ventricular fibrillation. Increased ventricular ectopic activity is probably the most common manifestation of digitalis toxic reaction. Initially a ventricular bigeminal rhythm develops, which is a relatively benign manifestation. Later, multiform ventricular ectopic beats may occur appearing singly or in groups, including ventricular tachycardia and ventricular fibrillation. Supraventricular tachycardias are commonly encountered, often at a rapid rate, associated with $2:1$ ventricular response. Conduction defects, up to and including complete AV block, are less commonly encountered. In patients who are in atrial fibrillation, the clinician should suspect digitalis intoxication when regular rhythm develops (other than conversion to sinus rhythm). A slow regular rhythm signifies complete AV block, whereas rapid regular rhythm signifies ectopic tachycardia or accelerated junctional rhythm. In patients in sinus rhythm, development of irregular rhythm is suspicious, particularly when it is due to ventricular ectopic activity. Supraventricular tachycardia or ventricular tachycardia may also develop in such patients.

Noncardiac digitalis toxic reaction is less ominous; nevertheless it may present confusing clinical pictures and escape recognition. Among such manifestations are gastrointestinal upsets, particularly anorexia and vomiting; cerebral manifestations (confusion, weakness, psychotic episodes are seen occasionally); and ocular disturbances (abnormalities in color vision, scotomata, and impaired vision are relatively commonly encountered).

It should be pointed out that the introduction of digitalis glycoside serum assays has been helpful in the prevention and early recognition of digitalis toxic reaction, yet the role of the serum assay is overrated: there is a wide overlap between the therapeutic and the toxic range of digoxin, so that in individual cases the knowledge of digoxin levels may be of limited value in guiding therapy. The important point is that the therapeutic effectiveness of digitalis bears no relationship to the serum level. Hence, the serum assay cannot be used as a guide for correct digitalis dosage.

Benefit of Digitalis

The benefit obtained from the slowing of ventricular rate in atrial fibrillation is clinically easily evident, often spectacular. Patients previously asymptomatic may develop acute cardiac failure from the rapid ventricular rate of uncontrolled atrial fibrillation, particularly when underlying cardiac disease is present (most frequently in mitral stenosis). Promptly slowing the ventricular rate usually restores full compensation. In patients who are in cardiac failure the onset of atrial fibrillation aggravates clinical manifestations of failure: digitalis is capable of restoring prefibrillation status. Cardiac failure in patients who are in established atrial fibrillation requires maintenance digitalis therapy. Even though other drugs (β-adrenergic blocking agents, calcium channel inhibitors) are capable of slowing the ventricular rate in atrial fibrillation, digitalis remains the drug of choice, provided the physician and the patient are fully aware of potential causes of digitalis intoxication.

Benefits of digitalis therapy in patients in sinus rhythm, dependent on the inotropic action of this drug, are more difficult to demonstrate. Strengthening of ventricular contraction can be shown by direct observation on muscle strips in animals and during cardiac operations in man. Acute digitalization in patients who are in cardiac failure produces an increase in cardiac output and a fall in atrial pressure in most but not all patients. However, two points are noteworthy. (1) Digitalis is a weak inotropic agent: hemodynamic responses to digitalis administration are lower than those of other inotropic agents or of vasodilating drugs. (2) The acute effects of digitalis appear to be blunted or even lost if observations extend over several hours.

Clinical studies in patients in cardiac failure and sinus rhythm produce contradictory results, particularly responses to discontinuation of digitalis maintenance. Although some hemodynamic or clinical deterioration when digitalis is stopped has been observed by some investigators, the majority of such studies have shown that discontinuation of digitalis does not produce adverse effects on patients in cardiac failure who are also managed by other interventions (e.g., diuretics). Considering these observations in the light of uncertainties regarding the correct dose of this drug, many investigators have expressed skepticism concerning the routine use of digitalis in patients in cardiac failure who are in sinus rhythm.

Clinical Use of Digitalis

Acute Heart Failure

Pump failure may develop abruptly in patients with impaired left ventricular function, particularly in the presence of compensatory hypertrophy. In the majority of patients a precipitating factor can be identified. Among those are onset of tachyarrhythmia, acute cardiac overload (e.g., hypertensive crisis, acute left ventricular valve incompetence), ischemia, overexertion, salt loading, and infection. As mentioned earlier, heart failure precipitated or aggravated by an uncontrolled ventricular rate in atrial fibrillation responds to administration of digitalis (usually intravenous digoxin or ouabain). In patients in acute cardiac failure who are in sinus rhythm, digitalis has serious disadvantages, discussed above. The use of diuretics and vasodilating agents is as a rule more effective; if additional inotropic stimulation is needed, synthetic catecholamines (dobutamine, dopamine) or newer inotropic agents (amrinone, milrinone) act faster and can be better controlled than digitalis.

In acute MI, reduced left ventricular performance is as a rule present, though overt heart failure develops only occasionally (usually in the presence of massive MI). Except in cases of heart failure developing in response to the onset of atrial fibrillation, digitalis therapy is to be avoided. In addition to the other disadvantages of digitalis, the proneness to ventricular ectopic activity in MI increases the risk of digitalis intoxication.

These same considerations apply to cardiogenic shock, a more severe variety of acute cardiac failure. Once recommended, digitalis is now by general consensus considered contraindicated in cardiogenic shock.

Chronic Cardiac Failure

Management of chronic heart failure in patients who are in sinus rhythm usually involves not only drug therapy but also regulation of life-style, with dietary adjustment and restriction of some activities. Recently, the importance of inotropic stimulation of the heart has been questioned on the basis of the hypothesis that reducing cardiac work load by limiting external activities and by using diuretics and vasodilating drugs constitutes a more physiologic approach than inotropic enhancement of the cardiac function. The question whether inotropic stimulation of the heart can maintain indefinitely improved cardiac performance has never been adequately tested and remains unanswered. As stated, several clinical studies have failed to show recurrence of cardiac failure on discontinuation of digitalis therapy. Both with initiation of therapy and with maintenance therapy, clinical improvement can easily be observed after administration of diuretics, but this is seldom apparent if the patient is treated with digitalis alone. The absence of clinically detectable improvement makes it impossible individually to adjust digitalis dosages. Thus, every patient receives the same dose of this drug. The opportunity to monitor the dose-effect relationship, so essential in management of atrial fibrillation, is not available in patients who are in sinus rhythm. The clinician has to appreciate that the recommended dose of digitalis based on averages is likely to benefit only some of his or her patients.

Even though digitalis is a weak inotropic agent, the possibility exists that some patients managed without digitalis may obtain additional benefit when digitalis is added. This hypothesis, however, has never been subjected to evaluation and remains merely a theoretical possibility. In "intractable" or "end-stage" heart failure conventional digitalisless therapy may not produce clinical improvement. Yet this stage is usually associated with severe myocardial damage and thus is particularly prone to digitalis intoxication.

Summary

Patients in cardiac failure caused by or associated with atrial fibrillation respond well to digitalis therapy aimed at slowing ventricular rate. The dose-effect relationship can be monitored and benefits are usually clearly detectable. With appropriate caution in avoiding digitalis intoxication, digitalis remains in such cases the first-line drug. Patients in cardiac failure who are in sinus rhythm are given digitalis for its inotropic effect, which is weak and clinically difficult, or even impossible, to detect. The potentially significant risk of digitalis intoxication probably overbalances the uncertain benefit of digitalis, especially since other therapeutic interventions, particularly diuretic and vasodilator therapy, are not only more effective but safer as well.

Bibliography

1. Cohn K, Selzer A, Kersh ES, et al: Variability of hemodynamic responses to acute digitalization in chronic cardiac failure due to cardiomyopthy and coronary artery disease. *Am J Cardiol* 1975; 35:461–468.

2. Flej TL, Gottlieb SH, Labana EG: Is digoxin really important in the treatment of compensated heart failure? *Am J Med* 1982; 73:244–250.
3. Gheorjiade M, Beller GA: Effect of discontinuing maintenance digoxin therapy in patients with ischemic heart disease and congestive heart failure in sinus rhythm. *Am J Cardiol* 1983; 151:1243–1250.
4. Lee DC, Johnson RA, Bingham JB, et al: Heart failure in outpatients: A randomized trial of digoxin versus placebo. *N Engl J Med* 1982; 305:696–705.
5. Selzer A: The use of digitalis in a cute myocardial infarction. *Prog Cardiovasc Dis* 1968; 10:518–528.
6. Selzer A: Digitalis in cardiac failure: Do benefits justify risks. *Arch Intern Med* 1981; 141:18–20.
7. Selzer A: Role of digoxin assay in patient management. *J Am Coll Cardiol* 1985; 5(suppl):106A–110A.
8. Smith TW, Antina EM, Friedman CM, et al: Digitalis glycoside: Mechanism and manifestations of toxicity. *Prog Cardiovasc Dis* 1981; Part I, 26:413–458; Part II, 26:495–540; Part III 27:21–56.
9. Smith TW, Haber E: Digitalis. *N Engl J Med* 1973; 289:945–952, 1010–1015, 1063–1072, 1125–1129.

Rebuttal: Affirmative
Barry H. Greenberg, M.D.

On perusing Dr. Selzer's manuscript, I was pleased to find that we had reached the same conclusion on many issues. Specifically, we agree that (1) digitalis is the drug of choice for controlling the ventricular response to atrial fibrillation in patients with CHF, (2) rapidly acting agents that can be easily titrated are preferable to digitalis for managing acute CHF, particularly when the patient is in sinus rhythm, and (3) digitalis toxic reaction is a clinically important problem that requires vigilance on the part of both the patient and the physician. We are also in agreement that the relationship between the dose of digitalis and the clinical response is inexact, so that monitoring serum levels is of limited value for the purpose of maximizing the cardiotonic effects of therapy. The major point over which we disagree is whether or not digitalis should be used to treat chronic CHF in patients who are in normal sinus rhythm. Dr. Selzer questions whether the benefits of digitalis therapy outweigh the risks and he suggests that comparable improvement may be obtained by agents with lesser risk.

If digitalis were a completely nontoxic drug, there would be little controversy about whether or not to give it to patients with CHF. However, serious and even life-threatening consequences of digitalis toxic reaction do occur in clinical practice. Furthermore, it is well known that the therapeutic-toxic ratio of digitalis is relatively low. Despite this fact, the incidence of serious cardiac arrhythmias or conduction abnormalities caused by digitalis has diminished considerably over the past two decades. There are several reasons for this favorable turn of events. The widespread availability of an assay to determine serum digitalis levels has been of value in confirming the presence of toxic reaction in suspected cases. It has also been helpful in titrating the dose of drug within a range where cardiac function is likely to be improved but the risk of toxic reaction is relatively low. This is especially relevant to the management of patients with renal dysfunction, since digoxin, the most commonly used digitalis preparation, is cleared by the kidney, and empirical determination of the optimal dose may be difficult in this setting. In addition, physician awareness of the high incidence of digitalis toxic reaction during the 1960s and early 1970s seems to have resulted in a more cautious approach to the use of this drug in general practice.

Although the potential for digitalis intoxication cannot be dismissed, it has become clear that careful surveillance can at least minimize this problem. On the other hand, the potential benefits of digitalis therapy are considerable provided that the drug is given in the appropriate clinical setting. Congestive heart failure is a syndrome characterized by reduced cardiac output and increased ventricular filling pressures. It may result from a variety of causes, and, as I have already discussed, the administration of digitalis to all patients with symptoms of heart failure will result in clinical improvement in only some. It is extremely important to determine whether or not left ventricular systolic pump function is impaired before initiating digitalis therapy. Treatment of noncardiac dyspnea and fatigue with digitalis will be a fruitless exercise. Similarly, when CHF is secondary to abnormal diastolic function or acute myocardial ischemia, treatment with digitalis will rarely be helpful. These points have been proved time and time again in clinical practice and they are the reason why many of the patients who were included in the studies alluded to by Dr. Selzer failed to show any evidence of clinical deterioration when digitalis was withdrawn. However, the large subset of patients with CHF due to left ventricular dysfunction have a reasonable likelihood of experiencing both hemodynamic and clinical improvement with digitalis.

The other point raised by Dr. Selzer is that diuretics, vasodilators, and some of the newer inotropic agents may be more effective in treating patients with chronic CHF. I am unaware of any published data from a well-controlled clinical trial that demonstrate the superiority of any of these agents compared with digitalis. In addition, each of these alternative approaches has its own attendant side effects and limitations. Diuretic agents play an important and well-deserved role in the treatment of patients with CHF. They are most useful in reducing ventricular filling pressures and treating the signs and symptoms of pulmonary and systemic congestion. Although diuretics may lead to some increase in cardiac output by virtue of their ability to reduce left ventricular systolic wall stress, myocardial ischemia, or the amount of mitral regurgitation (through improved valve leaflet coaption in a smaller ventricle), they generally don't have a major effect on forward flow. In fact, continued diuresis of the patient who is on the ascending limb of the Frank-Starling curve will result in an unwanted reduction in cardiac output, which may precipitate signs and symptoms of systemic hypoperfusion. Diuretics also have many unwanted secondary effects, the most important of which is their propensity to cause electrolyte abnormalities. Patients with CHF are at high risk of sudden cardiac death due to ventricular arrhythmias. Hypokalemia, which is commonly seen with many of the diuretic agents that are currently used, can increase the likelihood of this feared event.

The vasodilator drugs and newer inotropic agents have received a great deal of attention over the past decade. There is good evidence that some of the vasodilators such as the long-acting nitrates and the angiotensin-converting enzyme inhibitors can improve the clinical status of patients with heart failure. However, studies in which these agents are compared with digitalis are lacking. Furthermore, it is important to remember that not all patients respond favorably to vasodilator drugs and that the absolute improvement in exercise tolerance that has been demonstrated with vasodilators has been quite modest in most instances. Hypotension occurs with all vasodilators, and although this side effect is usually without clinical consequence it may, on occasion, be life-threatening. Other side effects of varying severity have been reported with the individual vasodilator drugs. Consequently, it is my feeling that, in most instances, vasodilators should be added to the therapeutic regimen of patients who are still symptomatic or who have limited exercise capacity while being treated with digitalis and diuretics. As mentioned in my position paper, good evidence of a beneficial clinical response with the newer inotropic drugs is lacking, and none of these drugs has been approved for the long-term management of patients with CHF.

The properties of an ideal drug for the treatment of CHF should include (1) a high likelihood of producing clinical improvement with a low risk of toxic reaction, (2) a long half-life so that infrequent dosing is possible, and (3) a predictable relationship between dose, serum concentration, and clinical effects. It is clear that none of the available agents fulfills all of these criteria. However, the demonstrated beneficial clinical effects of digitalis, the advantage of a daily dosing regimen, and the low cost lead me to the conclusion that it would be advisable to continue using this drug in the therapeutic regimen of patients with CHF due to left ventricular myocardial dysfunction.

Rebuttal: Negative

Arthur Selzer, M.D.

Dr. Greenberg and I are in agreement on most points. Differences of opinion lie primarily in the interpretation of available data and their clinical applications.

I agree that the pharmacologic properties of digitalis (inotropic, dromotropic, pressor, and venopressor effects) should be useful in controlling cardiac failure. But are they, in the light of the complex interaction of various hemodynamic and humoral factors, capable of overriding effects of digitalis? The answer is not available.

I agree that studies dealing with the clinical and hemodynamic efficacy of digitalis have produced contradictory results, and that the design of most studies leaves much to be desired. But is there a reason to consider positive results more reliable than negative ones, particularly since there are more studies showing negative rather than positive results? Two studies are singled out as convincing: those by Arnold et al. and Lee et al. Arnold's study deals with hemodynamic deterioration in patients in whom digitalis was discontinued. These changes are very small indeed: cardiac output at rest fell from 2.4 to 2.1 L/min/sq m, during exercise from 3.4 to 3.1 L/min/sq m. Wide variability of responses was found in individual cases. How significant is such a change, particularly in the light of growing awareness that the relationship between hemodynamic findings and clinical performance is poor?

Both Arnold's and Lee's studies show that only a little over one half of patients treated with digitalis performed better clinically with rather than without the drug. I prefer to interpret these findings as evidence for variability and unreliability of digitalis as an inotropic agent, rather than speculate why patients failed to respond to digitalis, especially since so many other studies failed to show any clinical difference between periods with and without digitalis. One should furthermore ask why it is so difficult to demonstrate significant clinical and hemodynamic improvement after administration of digitalis, when it is so easy to show often spectacular improvement after administration of diuretics or vasodilators in patients with cardiac failure.

The principal point at issue in this discussion is the use of digitalis as a first-line agent in treating patients with heart failure who are in sinus rhythm. The clinician should consider in the decision-making process the following points. (1) Milder forms of cardiac failure can, as a rule, be satisfactorily controlled by diuretic therapy. Nobody knows whether the addition of digitalis offers further advantages, yet it is generally recognized that by using digitalis, patients are subjected to a remote but real risk that somewhere along the line they may develop digitalis intoxication. (2) In severe cardiac failure diuretic therapy alone is usually inadequate. In considering other drugs it should be pointed out that we do not know how often digitalis is helpful, but we do know that most patients respond well to vasodilator therapy.

I do not deny that, in some cases with therapy-resistant cardiac failure, digitalis is worth trying, but I oppose the routine administration of this drug in treating patients in sinus rhythm who develop heart failure.

Editor's Comments
Nicholas J. Fortuin, M.D.

Drs. Greenberg and Selzer have covered succinctly the relevant recent literature and stated clearly their personal views about this important topic. Clinicians have for years blithely administered digitalis to patients with heart failure with little critical understanding of the proper use of the drug or its efficacy. As Dr. Greenberg points out, many patients with "heart failure" may not have heart disease at all or may have dysfunction of the heart that would not improve as a result of inotropic stimulation. Hence, many patients who receive the drug will not show improvement in functional status. This is particularly true of those with diastolic dysfunction (usually associated with ventricular hypertrophy or infiltrative processes), mechanical abnormalities (i.e., valvular dysfunction), or MI. This understanding emphasizes the point that it is absolutely essential for the physician to define as well as possible the cardiac abnormality that is responsible for abnormal fluid retention. Digitalis preparations are likely to be beneficial only when the left ventricle is dilated and there are demonstrable abnormalities of systolic function. How important this drug is in such a situation remains unclear. Dr. Selzer argues that the potency of digitalis as an inotropic agent is mild and that the use of potent diuretics and afterload-reducing agents renders the drug's contribution to the management of the patient with heart failure minimal. Dr. Greenberg feels differently, noting that digitalis glycosides are the only available agents that act to directly improve myocardial contractility. Both authors agree that the low therapeutic-toxic ratio of the drug makes it mandatory that its use be carefully monitored. Digitalis toxic reaction can be a subtle but formidable problem, which has often been unrecognized in the past. Clearly, increased awareness of the problem and the monitoring of serum levels have reduced its incidence.

I share Dr. Selzer's skepticism about digitalis, but I would agree with Dr. Greenberg that in the properly selected patient, digitalis does add an important therapeutic advantage. We all agree that in the patient with atrial fibrillation, digitalis is the drug of first choice for controlling the ventricular response.

Potassium Maintenance in Hypertensive Patients Receiving Diuretics Is Indicated in All Cases

Chapter Editor: H. Verdain Barnes, M.D.

Affirmative: Kim Goldenberg, M.D.
Associate Professor and Director, General
Internal Medicine Division, Department of
Medicine, Wright State University School of
Medicine, Dayton, Ohio

Negative: John F. Setaro, M.D.
Westchester Hypertension Foundation
Fellow, Department of Medicine, Yale
University School of Medicine, New Haven,
Connecticut

Henry R. Black, M.D.
Associate Professor of Medicine, Department
of Medicine, Yale University School of
Medicine, New Haven, Connecticut

Marvin Moser, M.D.
Clinical Professor of Medicine, Department
of Internal Medicine, Yale University School
of Medicine, New Haven, Connecticut

Debates in Medicine 1:138–165, 1988
©1988, Year Book Medical Publishers, Inc.
0887-218X/88/01-138-165-$04.00

Affirmative
Kim Goldenberg, M.D.

If hypertensive patients, treated with a potassium-wasting diuretic, become hypokalemic (serum potassium level ≤3.5 mEq/L) or decrease their potassium levels by more than 0.5 mEq/L from baseline, they should also receive a potassium-sparing diuretic. Potassium-wasting diuretics produce hypokalemia in up to 40% of patients, and the extent of potassium depression usually cannot be predicted for an individual patient. It is important to examine whether hypokalemia needs to be treated since there are up to 59 million hypertensive patients in this country, many of whom, if treated with medication, are given potassium-wasting as well as -sparing diuretics.

Few would argue that the potential untoward consequences of severe hypokalemia (potassium level <3.0 mEq/L) should be prevented, such as abnormal changes in carbohydrate, protein, and fat metabolism and structural as well as functional changes in the renal, neuromuscular, and cardiovascular systems. The extent to which a potassium level in the range of 3.0 to 4.0 mEq/L can produce some of these changes, especially cardiac arrhythmias and sudden death, is not clear. This uncertainty and controversy is highlighted by several large and small clinical trials in which hypokalemia and/or diuretics have been implicated in the pathogenesis of ventricular ectopia and sudden death.

The variation in the extent of hypokalemia that has been reported in different clinical trials is due to a number of potential factors that may have a major influence on potassium levels but are not usually controlled, such as diet (a low-sodium diet may correct hypokalemia, even in patients with primary aldosteronism), fecal excretion (use of laxatives is common, especially in the elderly), and intracellular shifts of potassium (diuretics may produce a metabolic alkalosis). In particular, intracellular potassium shifts may change the serum potassium level without affecting the total-body potassium level. At our institution, in patients who previously participated in the Multiple Risk Factor Intervention Trial (MRFIT), the measurement of total-body potassium level was limited by the precision of standard radioisotope techniques. For example, a 200 to 300 mEq/L loss of potassium may not have been detected. Thus, the measurements of blood and whole-body potassium changes usually do not correlate well, and there is no simple, inexpensive procedure for assessing the degree to which serum potassium represents total-body potassium or cellular potassium in critical organs of interest, such as the heart.

Even with our limited understanding of the pathophysiologic significance of mild hypokalemia and its effect on total-body potassium level and the heart, there is general agreement that there are certain subsets of patients for whom hypokalemia should be assiduously avoided. For example, those patients taking digitalis who are also hypokalemic have a definite increased risk of pathologic arrhythmias. These patients may more easily develop cardiac toxic reaction because both hypokalemia and digitalis inhibit the active sodium pump, which is responsible for transmembrane electrolyte balance. How many other subsets of patients should have their hypokalemia routinely treated, or should all hypertensive patients be considered at increased risk of untoward cardiac events from mild hypokalemia induced by diuretics? These questions were addressed, in part, by a number of studies that were originally designed to determine the effect of antihypertensive medication on mortality.

The MRFIT was designed to evaluate the impact of treatment on reducing three major risk factors for coronary artery disease: hypercholesterolemia, cigarette smoking, and diastolic blood pressure. Two randomized groups were compared: a special intervention (SI) group (counseling and antihypertensive medication) vs. a usual care (UC) group (private physician offices). There was no statistical difference in coronary mortality, perhaps because both groups were susceptible to extra care and education. For example, physicians in the UC group were well aware that their patients had been designated as high risk by a regional MRFIT center. Subsequent subgroup analysis revealed an unexpected result: patients receiving diuretics had over a threefold relative risk of coronary mortality if their baseline ECGs were abnormal. The diuretics used in the study, hydrochlorothiazide and chlorthalidone, were found to produce hypokalemia in a significant number of these patients. Thus, diuretics were considered to be responsible for the increased mortality. However, it was not retrospectively possible to explain the lack of a consistent relationship between the diuretic dosages, extent of hypokalemia, and coronary mortality.

The unexpected finding in the MRFIT, of diuretic-related coronary mortality, stimulated investigators in two other trials, the Hypertension Detection and Follow-up Program (HDFP) and the Oslo trial, to analyze their data retrospectively in a manner similar to the MRFIT. The HDFP was designed to evaluate the ability of antihypertensive medication to decrease mortality in hypertensive patients, especially those with mild hypertension. Two groups were compared: a stepped care (counseling and free medication with provision of transportation to the center) vs. a referred care (UC) group. Overall there was about a one-fifth reduced mortality in the stepped compared with the referred care group and a similar reduction in the subset with mild hypertension. These results may have been attributable, as in the MRFIT, to education as well as medication. Subsequent subgroup analysis of patients with an abnormal ECG, who were receiving the higher doses of diuretic, showed an increase in coronary mortality. This difference did not achieve statistical significance, however, due to the relatively small number of patients as compared with the number of patients in the MRFIT.

The Oslo trial was designed to evaluate the effect of antihypertensive medication on decreasing mortality in hypertensive male patients below 50 years of age whose diastolic blood pressure was under 110 mm Hg on entry into the study. Two randomized groups were compared: a treated (hydrochlorothiazide, with methyldopa or propranolol added as necessary to achieve target blood pressure) vs. an untreated group. There was no reduced morbidity or mortality in patients with a diastolic blood pressure under 100 mm Hg in either group but over a twofold decrease in cardiovascular morbidity in the treated vs. untreated groups. Subsequent subgroup analysis of patients with an abnormal ECG, on diuretic therapy, showed an increase in coronary mortality that again did not reach statistical significance due to the relatively small number of patients. Taken together, the implications of the MRFIT, HDFP, and Oslo trial, flawed in part by retrospective subgroup analysis, suggest that diuretic treatment, often associated with hypokalemia, could increase the risk of coronary mortality and sudden death in patients with an abnormal baseline ECG.

Although an abnormal ECG might be sufficient to galvanize some physicians into attempting to correct diuretic-induced hypokalemia, a related and equally important concern regards the induction or exacerbation of ventricular ectopy, which may be a precursor to sudden death. Since ventricular ectopy is related, in part, to the state of the cellular transmembrane potential, the concentrations of extracellular and intracellular potassium are important. At our institution, patients from the MRFIT, who were receiving hydrochlorothiazide or chlorthalidone, did not show any significant changes in intracellular potassium levels that were dependent on the diuretic dose or on the extent of hypokalemia. However, the thiazide diuretics did decrease extracellular potassium levels. These results, found at our and other institutions, may be important because a transmembrane difference in potassium concentration can hyperpolarize the cell membrane and prolong conduction. This potential for ventricular ectopic activity (VEA) combined with a significant risk in hypertensives, most of whose disease is not well controlled, for left ventricular hypertrophy and/or coronary artery disease encompasses a major subset of hypertensive patients.

In the MRFIT, patients who were treated with diuretics had a significantly greater number of ventricular premature beats. Smaller studies have revealed conflicting results regarding the association of diuretic-induced hypokalemia and VEA. In 1981, Holland et al. showed that about one fifth of patients with hypokalemia developed new high-grade arrhythmias (Lown grades 3 through 5 VEA) after the mean potassium level decreased from 4.0 to 3.0 mEq/L. Subsequently, they and others showed that, on the average, about one third of patients developed high-grade arrhythmias with mild hypokalemia (the fall in potassium level ranged from 4.1 to 3.2 mEq/L). However, the patients in one series were restricted to the elderly and in another series had no initial baseline monitoring of ECG activity.

No increase in serious arrhythmias occurred in a number of other series.

The largest number of patients in these other series, however, only had a small mean potassium level change, from 4.1 to 3.8 mEq/L, and these studies were conducted without exercise induction.

Since exercise-related arrhythmias may portend a more serious prognosis than rest-related arrhythmias, some investigators have examined ventricular activity with exercise in diuretic-treated patients. Hollifield showed an increased incidence of exercise-related VEA in patients who were hypokalemic receiving diuretics. With hydrochlorothiazide therapy the number of low-grade arrhythmias increased, but, more importantly, the increases were moderately correlated with decreases in levels of both serum potassium and magnesium. Since ventricular arrhythmia often precedes sudden cardiac death, the increased incidence of VEA, both with and without exercise, is of some concern.

Sudden cardiac death was the major terminal event for a thiazide-treated group in the Veterans Administration Cooperative Study. Twice as many deaths occurred in the drug-treated group (reserpine and chlorthalidone) as in the placebo-treated group. The mean serum potassium level changed from 4.3 to 3.5 mEq/L. Although the change in mean potassium levels did not produce severe hypokalemia, a relative fall of 0.8 mEq/L had occurred.

The risk of ventricular ectopia, especially ventricular fibrillation, during a myocardial infarction was studied in normokalemic and hypokalemic patients by Nordrehaug and von der Lippe. In a sizeable number of patients with hypokalemia, about one fifth developed ventricular fibrillation as compared with less than half that amount in a larger group of normokalemic patients (Fig 1). The risk of fibrillation increased with both hypokalemia and hyperkalemia. In the latter, hypotension, shock, and acidosis may have been precipitants. In other studies mortality in the first 24 hours was increased if hypokalemia was present on admission. A number of small, less well-controlled trials have reported data on patients who were hypokalemic, but not necessarily receiving diuretics, who also had an increased incidence of ventricular fibrillation.

Patients with a myocardial infarction may be at particular risk for hypokalemia because of an epinephrine-mediated stimulation of their sodium pump at the β_2-receptor site. Increased pump activity, transfer of potassium into the cell, and a subsequent decline in serum potassium has been experimentally shown. Struthers et al. have clinically demonstrated, in healthy volunteers, that infusing "stress" levels of adrenaline leads to a rapid diminution of potassium level. Serum potassium level fell by up to 1.0 mEq/L in both thiazide-treated subjects and normal controls (Fig 2).

Correction of a low serum potassium level in thiazide-treated patients usually requires a consideration of any potential concomitant magnesium deficiency because hypomagnesemia contributes to refractory potassium depletion. About 40% of patients with hypokalemia may have coexisting hypomagnesemia, and a depletion of both cations is related to the devel-

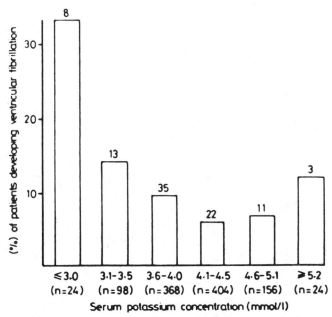

FIG 1.
Number and percentage of patients developing ventricular fibrillation in relation to serum potassium concentration. Of the 122 patients with hypokalemia, 17.2% developed ventricular fibrillation compared with 7.5% of the 952 normokalemic patients (*P* <.01). (From Nordrehaug JE, von der Lippe G: Hypokalaemia and ventricular fibrillation in acute myocardial infarction. *Br Heart J* 1983; 50:525. Reproduced by permission.)

opment of cardiac arrhythmias. In patients receiving thiazide diuretics, with potassium and magnesium deficiencies, the replacement therapy of both cations reduces ventricular ectopy to a greater extent than does replacing potassium alone.

Giving intravenous magnesium to patients with a myocardial infarction has reduced both initial mortality and serious arrhythmias. The detailed mechanism by which hypomagnesemia produces arrhythmias (inhibition of the sodium pump and partial depolarization of the membrane) and by which it creates refractory depletion of potassium (decreased transfer of extracellular potassium into the cells) is not completely understood. However, the role of hypomagnesemia in arrhythmogenesis and in the treatment of refractory hypokalemia has recently been better appreciated. As is the case with potassium, serum levels of magnesium may not reflect the degree of magnesium deficit.

It is of interest and concern that a higher mortality in diuretic-treated

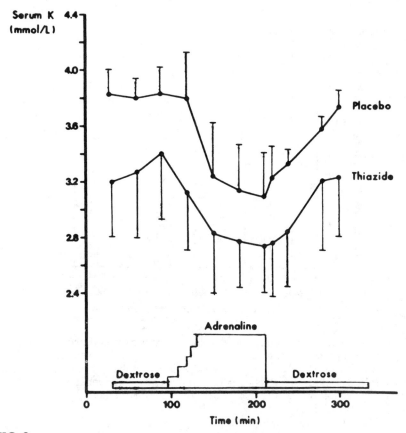

FIG 2.
Serum potassium (mean ± SD) during infusion of 5% dextrose, 0.06 μg/kg/min adrenaline, and 5% dextrose again in six patients after pretreatment with placebo or bendroflumethiazide (5 mg) for 7 days. (From Struthers AD, Whitesmith R, Reid JL: Prior thiazide diuretic treatment increases adrenaline-induced hypokaelemia. *Lancet* 1983; 1:1358. Reproduced by permission.)

patients from the MRFIT could not be explained by hypokalemia alone. In two centers from the MRFIT, diuretic-treated patients had mild reductions in magnesium levels, and in the Medical Research Council trial, increased ventricular ectopia was noted in thiazide-treated patients both with and without hypokalemia. The recent European Working Party trial, in hypertensive patients over 60 years old, showed that a combination of hydrochlorothiazide and triamterene (methyldopa was added as necessary to achieve target blood pressures) produced a major decrease in cardiac mortality and in myocardial infarction deaths when compared with placebo.

The frequency of sudden death also diminished. Since potassium-sparing diuretics, such as triamterene, are also known to spare magnesium, it is not difficult to perceive the potential benefit of preventing hypomagnesemia, a known arrhythmogenic condition.

In conclusion, hypokalemia should be treated in hypertensive patients receiving potassium-wasting diuretics to prevent the increased likelihood of cardiac arrhythmia and sudden death suggested, though not established, by numerous clinical trials. Since it is not possible to predict which patients will suffer a myocardial infarction and be particularly prone to the arrhythmogenic potential of stress- and/or diuretic-induced hypokalemia, patients with hypokalemia (serum potassium level ≤3.5 mEq/L) should be treated. Patients should also be treated if their potassium level falls by more than 0.5 mEq/L. This strategy would result in treating many to save a few, but that is precisely the strategy used in treating mild hypertension.

A potassium-sparing diuretic should be added, rather than replacement therapy, so that potential magnesium losses may also be prevented. Replacement of magnesium by supplements is not practical, palatable, or without side effects such as diarrhea. Similarly, although potassium supplements are now more palatable than in the past because of the advent of enteric coating, lack of compliance is still a problem for many patients. Risks of treatment are known to be small, with combined potassium-wasting and -sparing diuretics, if patients with known predispositions to hyperkalemia and hypermagnesemia are excluded, such as patients with renal insufficiency.

Given the widespread use of these combination diuretics (one of the most commonly prescribed medications) and the well-known compliance problems with supplements, it appears that the collective wisdom of many practicing physicians (to use combination diuretics) is the strategy most likely to benefit the patient and cause him or her the least harm. This strategy is consistent with the recommendations of the 1984 Joint National Committee on the Detection, Evaluation, and Treatment of High Blood Pressure. Whenever possible, however, the initiation of a potassium-wasting diuretic, before the addition of a potassium-sparing diuretic, should be combined with advice to the patient regarding dietary fortification with potassium, the substitution of sodium with potassium salts, and assurance of adequate amounts of magnesium in the diet.

Bibliography

1. European Working Party on High Blood Pressure in the Elderly: Mortality and morbidity results from the European Working Party on High Blood Pressure in the Elderly. *Lancet* 1985; 1:1349–1354.
2. Holland OB, Nixon JV, Kuhnert L: Diuretic induced ventricular ectopic activity. *Am J Med* 1981; 70:762–768.

3. Hollifield JW: Potassium and magnesium abnormalities: Diuretics and arrhythmias in hypertension. *Am J Med* 1984; 77(suppl):28–32.
4. Holme I, Helgeland A, Hjermann I, et al: Treatment of mild hypertension with diuretics: The importance of ECG abnormalities in the Oslo study and in MRFIT. *JAMA* 1984; 251:1298–1299.
5. Joint National Committee on Detection, Evaluation, and Treatment of High Blood Pressure: The 1984 report of the Joint National Committee on Detection, Evaluation, and Treatment of High Blood Pressure. *Arch Intern Med* 1984; 140:1045–1057.
6. Medical Research Council Working Party on Mild to Moderate Hypertension: Ventricular extrasystoles during thiazide treatment: Substudy of MRC mild hypertension trial. *Br Med J* 1983; 287:1249–1253.
7. Messerli FH, Ventura HO, Elizardi DJ, et al: Hypertension and sudden death: Increased ventricular ectopic activity in left ventricular hypertrophy. *Am J Med* 1984; 77:18–22.
8. Multiple Risk Factor Intervention Trial Research Group: Baseline rest electrocardiographic abnormalities, antihypertensive treatment, and mortality in the Multiple Risk Factor Intervention Trial. *Am J Cardiol* 1985; 55:1–15.

Negative
John F. Setaro, M.D., Henry R. Black, M.D., and Marvin Moser, M.D.

Controversy exists surrounding the use of potassium therapy, either as a potassium sparing diuretic or potassium supplementation, when thiazide diuretics are used to treat hypertension. Should such potassium maintenance therapy be used in all patients, only in those at high risk for arrhythmias, sudden death, or metabolic disturbances, or not at all?

The answer to this question assumes great importance because of the large numbers of patients treated with diuretics. These medications are simple to use and are effective as antihypertensive therapy. They have been the mainstay of treatment for nearly 30 years, especially in the United States. A dramatic decrease in stroke mortality over the past 15 years (50.2%) and a reduced incidence of renal and cardiac complications of hypertension attest to the benefits of widespread treatment, much of which has included diuretics.

Yet in the 1980s many authorities have questioned the wisdom of using diuretics as routine monotherapy. Their reasons have included concerns about electrolyte imbalance, coronary artery disease, and sudden death. Two large clinical trials of hypertension management, the MRFIT and the Oslo Study of Mild Hypertension, as well as several smaller studies, have raised the suspicion that diuretics, with attendant hypokalemia and possible risk of cardiac arrhythmias, may have, in fact, increased the risk of mortality from ischemic heart disease. This proposition deserves serious analysis for, if correct, it suggests that most patients receiving these agents may also need to receive potassium-sparing agents or routine potassium supplementation.

Hypokalemia and Thiazides

It is acknowledged that treatment with standard doses of a thiazide diuretic reduces serum potassium levels to the hypokalemic range (<3.5 mEq/L) in 20% to 30% of patients. Typically, a decrease in serum potassium level of 0.6 to 0.7 mEq/L occurs when 100 mg of hydrochlorothiazide or its equivalent is given. Approximately 5% of all patients treated will have significant hypokalemia (serum potassium level ≤3.0 mEq/L). Although some investigators have demonstrated a linear relationship between dosages of hydrochlorothiazide, serum potassium levels, and total-body potassium stores, others have reported that total-body potassium losses are quite small (200 mEq on average from a total-body pool of

3,500 mEq) in spite of diuretic-induced hypokalemia. It is important to recognize that many factors influence the serum levels of potassium. Aside from intake and thiazide-induced urinary losses, these include acid-base status, insulin deficiency, serum glucose, catecholamine excess, renal function, and degree of aldosterone secretion.

After reviewing the data on diuretic-induced hypokalemia and outcome of treatment, the Joint National Committee on the Detection, Evaluation, and Treatment of High Blood Pressure in 1984 stated that only some patients who receive diuretics need to be treated with potassium supplements or potassium-sparing agents. These patients include the elderly, persons on low-potassium diets, patients with pretreatment ectopia, those taking digitalis preparations, and patients with known ischemic heart disease. Are these conclusions reasonable or should these categories be expanded based on the results of studies that address the question of hypokalemia in the settings of left ventricular hypertrophy, baseline abnormalities in the ECG, and ventricular ectopia?

Left Ventricular Hypertrophy

Hypertensive patients with ECG-documented left ventricular hypertrophy have been shown to exhibit more high-grade ventricular ectopia than those without an increase in left ventricular muscle mass. This observation is consistent with conclusions drawn from the Framingham Heart Study, which suggest that subjects with evidence of left ventricular hypertrophy (determined by ECG) have a greater risk for sudden death. Together, these studies may have identified a group of hypertensives at greater risk for arrhythmias and in whom hypokalemia probably should be prevented. It would appear, therefore, that patients with left ventricular hypertrophy should be considered for potassium maintenance therapy. However, in a retrospective study of patients at the Glasgow High Blood Pressure Clinic published in 1986, no relationship was found between serum potassium level and mortality in patients with left ventricular hypertrophy, and Papademetriou and coworkers found no relationship between diuretic-induced hypokalemia and significant ectopia in their hypertensive patients with left ventricular hypertrophy. Clearly, further study is needed.

Abnormal Baseline ECGs

Several clinical trials have been analyzed to assess the relationship between thiazides, hypokalemia, and mortality in patients with organic heart disease as evidenced by abnormal baseline ECG. The MRFIT and the Oslo study suggested possible ill effects of diuretics in the setting of abnormal

ECGs, whereas the HDFP, the International Prospective Primary Prevention Study in Hypertension (IPPPSH), and the Glasgow series did not.

The MRFIT results originally called attention to the problem of ischemic heart disease and diuretic therapy. This was a long-term multicenter study, the aim of which was to determine whether patients would benefit from vigorous treatment designed to alter the three major cardiovascular risk factors. High-risk males were selected for the study on the basis of excessive cigarette smoking, elevated serum cholesterol level, and/or elevated diastolic blood pressure. Those chosen were randomized to an SI group (the "experimental" cohort) or a UC group (the intended "control" group), the latter to be treated by local practitioners who were, in fact, fully aware of the high-risk designation that their patients had received at the MRFIT centers. The overall results of the study revealed a nonsignificant reduction in coronary artery disease mortality in the SI group as compared with the UC group, although both groups experienced a marked decrease in the anticipated number of deaths. For example, it had been estimated that 442 subjects would die in the UC group during the study, yet only 260 deaths occurred. Possibly this happened because the control group's cholesterol levels had been reduced, blood pressure lowered, and smoking decreased to a greater degree than was originally anticipated. Physicians in the community and their patients had responded to the risk factor message. This low death rate made it impossible to discern statistically significant differences between the SI and UC groups; a larger sample size would have been needed to achieve sufficient statistical power. What was disturbing, however, was that hypertensive men with *any* resting pretreatment ECG abnormalities exhibited a higher mortality in the SI group.

Retrospective subgroup analysis showed that the excess mortality was mainly due to sudden death in the group with resting ECG abnormalities. This mortality was independent of baseline blood pressure or findings on exercise ECG. Actually, SI patients with abnormal stress test results had a lower mortality than comparable UC patients (Table 1).

In trying to explain these findings, the investigators performed further subgroup analyses. It was presumed that lower doses of diuretics, usually hydrochlorothiazide or chlorthalidone, had been administered in the UC group of patients although diuretics had been used for treatment in both the UC and SI patients (a higher percentage of SI patients received these agents). The MRFIT investigators hypothesized that patients with abnormal ECGs might have been harmed by the use of diuretics and that hypokalemia-induced arrhythmias contributed to the increased rate of sudden death seen in thiazide-treated hypertensives in the SI group.

Yet several inconsistencies have raised doubts about this interpretation of the data. (1) There was no correlation between mortality and diuretic dosage, nor did the potassium levels found on the visit before death correlate with fatal events. (2) A higher mortality was seen in patients treated with hydrochlorothiazide despite more hypokalemia in the patients receiv-

TABLE 1.
Five-Year Mortality: MRFIT vs. HDFP
Subgroups*

Resting ECG	MRFIT		HDFP	
	SI	**UC**	**Special Care**	**Referred Care**
Normal	15.8	20.7	33.7	47.3
Abnormal	29.2	17.7	57.9	75.3

*Per 1,000 patient-years.

ing chlorthalidone. (3) Patients in the SI group with abnormal baseline ECGs who received the higher dosages of chlorthalidone actually had lower mortality than those receiving lower dosages (Table 2).

Other criticisms focus on the all-inclusive definition of an abnormal ECG. This encompassed relatively mild changes such as an abnormal electrical axis, incomplete bundle-branch block, and nonspecific early repolarization changes as well as more serious abnormalities such as Q waves, left ventricular hypertrophy, and ventricular ectopia. Finally, and most importantly, UC subjects with abnormal ECGs had an *unexpectedly* low death

TABLE 2.
MRFIT: Mortality and Diuretic Dose

Diuretic Dose, mg	SI Group Mortality*	
	ECG Abnormal	**ECG Normal**
Chlorthalidone	3.31	2.08
<50	4.84	1.76
>50	1.84	2.37
Hydrochlorothiazide	7.61	2.21
<50	7.20	2.27
>50	8.01	2.55

*Per 1,000 patient-years.

rate and therefore a lower mortality than UC subjects with normal ECGs. This result differs from the findings of all other studies: it is the only one in which the death rates were lower for subjects with abnormal ECGs whether or not they received any treatment. If the ratio in this subgroup had been similar to that in other trials or to the other subgroups in this trial, there would be no need to postulate a diuretic-induced toxic reaction.

The MRFIT analysis is important because the results of this study have often been quoted to justify curtailing the use of diuretics as first-step monotherapy for high blood pressure or to promote the universal use of potassium supplements or sparing agents to avoid hypokalemia. Perhaps the problem of what to do with MRFIT can be summarized best by a quote from Grimm, one of the MRFIT investigators: "The MRFIT subgroup results could have occurred by chance; therefore the results are not definitive and should be interpreted with caution . . . A possible explanation is that a comparable UC subgroup experienced an unusually low coronary heart disease mortality.

Other studies, such as the Oslo Study of Mild Hypertension, are also quoted to suggest a link between thiazide therapy and coronary death. This study reported six deaths from coronary disease at the end of 5 years in the diuretic-treated group compared with only two in a control group. This difference failed to achieve significance. At 10-year follow-up, there were 14 deaths in the original treatment group compared with three in the control group, but no data were available relating to type of therapy or morbidity from the 5th to the 10th year. It is possible that a large number of control patients whose pressures had been high were placed on a specific medication regimen; on the other hand, many treated patients whose pressures were well regulated may have been taken off the treatment regimen. The Oslo authors have urged caution with the interpretation of their data.

On the other hand, the HDFP trial showed no increased mortality in hypertensive patients with resting ECG abnormalities while taking thiazides. In addition, the IPPPSH study failed to detect a relationship between sudden death and hypokalemia in thiazide-treated patients. Finally, a retrospective analysis in 1986 of nearly 2,000 patients followed up in the Glasgow High Blood Pressure Clinic indicated that mild hypokalemia was not a risk factor for death from ischemic heart disease; final recorded serum potassium values for those dying of ischemic heart disease were not significantly different compared with those of survivors (3.71 vs. 3.72 mEq/L, respectively).

Ventricular Ectopia

Several controlled studies have been done to look directly at the relationship of diuretic therapy to ventricular ectopia. Hollifield, Holland et al., and a 1985 Medical Research Council of Great Britain trial showed a possible link between diuretics and ventricular ectopia, and Caralis et al. demonstrated this as well, though only in older patients with organic heart disease. Yet Papademetriou et al., Madias et al., Lief et al., and another Medical Research Council trial failed to show a relationship between thiazides and ventricular arrhythmias.

In 1981, Hollifield and Slaton reported an increased frequency of ventricular ectopia during exercise testing of hypertensives treated with thiazide diuretics. Patients with known cardiac disease were excluded from this study. The subjects who developed arrhythmias or had significant increases in ectopia usually had *severe* hypokalemia (potassium level <3.0 mEq/L). Little difficulty occurred in patients with milder degrees of hypokalemia.

In 1984, Hollifield described hypokalemia in patients treated with up to 200 mg of hydrochlorothiazide daily. Yet those treated with 100 mg or less showed mean potassium values higher than or equal to 3.4 mEq/L. Premature ventricular contractions increased as serum potassium levels fell, though approximately only one per minute was recorded on a dose of 50 mg/day of hydrochlorothiazide. This study is important because, while it shows that *very high* doses of diuretics are associated with hypokalemia and ectopia, moderate doses appear to have little ill effect.

Other work that has suggested a connection between diuretic use and ventricular ectopia includes that of Holland et al. in 1981. They showed that, in seven of 21 patients who had severe hypokalemia (mean serum potassium ≤3.0 mEq/L), more frequent and severe ectopia occurred after treatment with 100 mg of hydrochlorothiazide. Since Holland et al. excluded all patients with baseline ventricular ectopia (greater than six premature ventricular contractions per hour), any ectopia that occurred was blamed on diuretics and hypokalemia. With such low pretreatment levels of ectopia, the probability of finding heightened frequency of posttreatment ectopia was greatly enhanced, simply by chance. Caralis et al. studied two groups of patients: one was an older group with organic heart disease and the second a younger cohort without disease. They noted that the patients with heart disease receiving thiazides had an increased frequency and severity of ventricular arrhythmias, which were abolished after correction of hypokalemia. Data from this study suggest that diuretic-induced hypokalemia may lead to arrhythmias in patients with organic heart disease.

Finally, a clinical trial often cited as evidence implicating diuretics in arrhythmias is that of the Medical Research Council of Great Britain. Compared with a group receiving placebos, hypertensive patients receiving long-term thiazide therapy exhibited an increase in ventricular ectopia. Yet this study was uncontrolled in that no pretreatment baseline ECG monitoring had been performed. Moreover, in the treated group with increased ectopia, no correlation was observed between arrhythmias and serum potassium values.

There have been major problems, therefore, with the studies cited above. In general, these studies actually have not proved the harmful effects of thiazides and the relationship of diuretic-induced hypokalemia and arrhythmias. There are an equal number of negative studies that fail to demonstrate a relationship.

For example, in another Medical Research Council study, shorter in duration yet well controlled with pretreatment and posttreatment ECG monitoring, no difference was noted in the prevalence of arrhythmias in placebo- vs. thiazide-treated patients, in spite of the appearance of some hypokalemia (to the degree usually observed in the average patient).

Several studies by Papademetriou and colleagues also were unable to demonstrate a relationship between thiazides, hypokalemia, and arrhythmias. The first, published in 1983, showed that, in uncomplicated hypertensives treated with thiazides, correction of diuretic-induced hypokalemia did not suppress atrial or ventricular ectopic beats. In a controlled study in 1985, his group found that thiazide treatment did not increase ventricular arrhythmias in patients with or without left ventricular hypertrophy (Table 3).

TABLE 3.
Ectopia in Subjects With and Without LVH Before and After Treatment With Hydrochlorothiazide*

	Patients With LVH (n = 18)		Patients Without LVH (n = 13)	
	Before	After	Before	After
Plasma potassium, mEq/L	4.1 ± 0.3	3.3 ± 0.4	4.1 ± 0.3	3.4 ± 0.5
Average PVCs/hr	5.7 ± 9.9	7.1 ± 16.6	4.3 ± 8.0	5.2 ± 8.9
Total couplets	29	13	0	1
Total episodes VT	4	0	1	1
Average grade/hr†	0.77 ± 0.77	0.78 ± 0.83	0.45 ± 0.50	0.49 ± 0.62

*From Papademetriou V, Price M, Notargiacomo A, et al: Effect of diuretic therapy on ventricular arrhythmias in hypertensive patients with or without left ventricular hypertrophy. *Am Heart J* 1985; 110:595–599. Reproduced by permission. LVH indicates left ventricular hypertrophy; PVC, premature ventricular contractions; VT, ventricular tachycardia.
†Modified Lown classification.

Madias et al. have also demonstrated that hypokalemia produced by a short course of diuretics did not result in ventricular ectopia in patients who had none before treatment. Ectopia did not increase in patients who exhibited arrhythmias *before* treatment was inaugurated (Madias et al. and Papademetriou et al. did not exclude subjects with pretreatment ectopia). Lief et al. also failed to demonstrate increased ectopia in diuretic-treated subjects.

Hypokalemia and Infarction

The problem of hypokalemia in the setting of myocardial infarction is important because hypertensives are known to be at risk for atherosclerotic coronary artery disease. It is necessary to know whether their antihypertensive therapy would predispose them to malignant arrhythmias should a coronary event occur.

The stress induced by myocardial infarction causes a release of catecholamines into the plasma, where they act to drive potassium into cells. This, of course, results in decreased serum potassium levels. Struthers et al. demonstrated that when catecholamines were infused into subjects pretreated with thiazides, the serum potassium fell to a greater level than in those pretreated with placebo. Several studies have reported an increase in significant arrhythmias in low potassium states during the first 24 hours following an infarction. This occurs regardless of whether or not a patient has received a diuretic. Based on available data, it is impossible to judge whether pretreatment with a diuretic increases the risk of serious arrhythmias. The evidence connecting thiazides, hypokalemia, and arrhythmia in the setting of infarction is circumstantial at best. It is well known that, at least in patients without coronary vascular disease, increased catecholamines may cause major potassium shifts into skeletal muscle with only minor effects on myocardial cell concentrations. Thus, it is difficult to postulate harmful effects of this type on patients with normal cardiac function.

Conclusion

An overview of the above studies suggests that diuretics are safe and effective and that the mild degree of hypokalemia usually seen with these agents is well tolerated in the majority of uncomplicated hypertensive patients. The hypothesis that ventricular arrhythmias and the incidence of sudden death are increased significantly in patients receiving diuretics has not been confirmed. The risk appears to be small, and the studies showing risk are generally inadequate to offer proof. Thus, *routine* administration of potassium supplements or potassium-sparing therapy in all patients at the initiation of treatment is unwarranted.

Recommendations for Maintenance Therapy

In which subcategories might potassium maintenance or potassium-sparing therapy be appropriate? They include (1) those patients with organic heart disease, especially ischemic disease, who should receive such therapy since possible benefit exists provided that careful attention is paid to serum potassium levels to avoid hyperkalemia; (2) patients taking digitalis preparations, who should be given potassium maintenance treatment since a definite demonstrated correlation between diuretic-induced hypokalemia and ventricular arrhythmias exists in conjunction with digitalis administration; (3) patients who exhibit high levels of pretreatment ectopia; (4) diabetics, especially the non–insulin-dependent type, who need to have potassium levels monitored carefully and probably should receive potassium supplementation or potassium-sparing agents (in these patients, basal insulin secretion may be suppressed by hypokalemia, thereby aggravating problems with blood glucose control); to avoid hyperkalemia, renal function must be monitored carefully in patients with diabetic nephropathy and concomitant hypoaldosteronism if potassium maintenance therapy is carried out; (5) the elderly, whose diets may be deficient in potassium, and thus probably need maintenance therapy; renal function must be monitored closely (in this age group glomerular filtration rate may be significantly reduced though serum creatinine level is normal or only mildly increased); (6) alcoholics, who often are hypokalemic and hypomagnesemic and are likely to benefit from potassium maintenance therapy; (7) those at risk of hepatic coma, a condition that tends to occur more readily and with greater severity in the potassium-deficient state; these patients merit maintenance regimens; and finally, (8) those patients who become markedly hypokalemic (potassium level <3.2 mEq/L) or who demonstrate signs of hypokalemia (weakness and cramps) and thus need potassium maintenance. It is probably easier and less expensive in most instances to use a combination diuretic–potassium-sparing agent than to employ potassium supplements plus a thiazide diuretic.

Choice of Agents and Doses

The diuretic type and manner in which it is prescribed may govern whether hypokalemia will be a problem. Presumably because of its shorter duration of action, hydrochlorothiazide exerts less of an effect on potassium than metolazone and chlorthalidone; the use of either of these agents may require concurrent potassium supplementation. The least dose that is effective should be prescribed, since potassium loss is dose related. We recommend lower maximum doses of diuretics and favor 25 to 50 mg/day of hydrochlorothiazide for most patients. A moderately sodium-restricted diet is advised. This may help to reduce potassium loss in conjunction with its possible beneficial effect on arterial blood pressure.

Is potassium maintenance therapy safe? Lawson showed it to be safe in an ambulatory population, and the European Working Party on High Blood Pressure in the Elderly used a combination thiazide and potassium-sparing agent with good clinical results and less than a 0.2 mEq/L depression in serum potassium values.

Most hypertensives do not need potassium maintenance therapy. In the selected patients who do, low doses of diuretics and close observation to avoid hyperkalemia will ensure good results. Thus, with some modification, we concur with the 1984 Joint National Committee recommendations.

Bibliography

GENERAL
1. Joint National Committee on Detection, Evaluation, and Treatment of High Blood Pressure: The 1984 report of the Joint National Committee on Detection, Evaluation, and Treatment of High Blood Pressure. Arch Intern Med 1984; 140:1045–1057.
2. Moser M: Historical perspective on the management of hypertension. Am J Med 1986; 80(suppl 5B):1–11.
3. Moser M: The diuretic dilemma and the management of mild hypertension. J Clin Hypertens 1986; 2:195–202.

DIURETICS AND HYPOKALEMIA
4. European Working Party on High Blood Pressure in the Elderly: Mortality and morbidity results from the European Working Party on High Blood Pressure in the Elderly. Lancet 1985; 1:1349–1354.
5. Kaplan NM: Our appropriate concern about hypokalemia. Am J Med 1984; 77:1–4.
6. Lawson DH: Adverse reactions to potassium chloride. Q J Med 1974; 43:433–440.
7. Tannen RL: Diuretic-induced hypokalemia. Kidney Int 1985; 28:988–1000.

LEFT VENTRICULAR HYPERTROPHY
8. Messerli FH, Ventura HO, Elizardi DJ, et al: Hypertension and sudden death: Increased ventricular ectopic activity in left ventricular hypertrophy. Am J Med 1984; 77:18–22.
9. Papademetriou V, Price M, Notargiacomo A, et al: Effect of diuretic therapy on ventricular arrhythmias in hypertensive patients with or without left ventricular hypertrophy. Am Heart J 1985; 110:595–599.
10. Robertson JWK, Isles CG, Brown I, et al: Mild hypokalemia is not a risk factor in treated hypertensives. J Hypertens 1986; 4:603–608.

BASELINE ABNORMAL ECGS
11. Atwood JE, Gardin JM: Diuretics, hypokalemia, and ventricular ectopy: The controversy continues. Arch Intern Med 1985; 145:1185–1187.

12. Holme I, Helgeland A, Hjermann I, et al: Treatment of mild hypertension with diuretics: The importance of ECG abnormalities in the Oslo study and in MRFIT. *JAMA* 1984; 251:1298–1299.
13. International Prospective Primary Prevention Study in Hypertension. *J Hypertens* 1985; 3:1–13.
14. Hypertension Detection and Follow-up Program Cooperative Research Group: The effect of antihypertensive drug treatment on mortality in the presence of resting electrocardiographic abnormalities at baseline: The HDFP experience. *Circulation* 1984; 70:996–1003.
15. Kuller LH, Hulley SB, Cohen JD, et al: Unexpected effects of treating hypertension in men with electrocardiographic abnormalities: A critical analysis. *Circulation* 1986; 73:114–123.
16. Multiple Risk Factor Intervention Trial Research Group: Multiple Risk Factor Intervention Trial: Risk factor changes and mortality results. *JAMA* 1982; 248:1465–1477.
17. Multiple Risk Factor Intervention Trial Research Group: Baseline rest electrocardiographic abnormalities, antihypertensive treatment, and mortality in the Multiple Risk Factor Intervention Trial. *Am J Cardiol* 1985; 55:1–15.
18. Moser M: Clinical trials and their effect on medical therapy: The Multiple Risk Factor Intervention Trial. *Am Heart J* 1984; 107:616–618.

VENTRICULAR ECTOPIA
19. Caralis PV, Materson BJ, Perez-Stable E: Potassium and diuretic-induced ventricular arrhythmias in ambulatory hypertensive patients. *Miner Electrolyte Metab* 1984; 10:148–154.
20. Holland OB, Nixon JV, Kuhnert L: Diuretic induced ventricular ectopic activity. *Am J Med* 1981; 70:762–768.
21. Hollifield JW, Slaton PE: Thiazide diuretics, hypokalemia, and cardiac arrhythmias. *Acta Scand Med* 1981; 647(suppl):67–73.
22. Hollifield JW: Potassium and magnesium abnormalities: Diuretics and arrhythmias in hypertension. *Am J Med* 1984; (suppl):28–32.
23. Lief PD, Beligon I, Mates J, et al: Diuretic-induced hypokalemia does not cause ventricular ectopy in uncomplicated essential hypertension, abstracted. *Kidney Int* 1984; 24:203.
24. Madias JE, Madias NE, Gavras HP: Nonarrhythmogenicity of diuretic-induced hypokalemia: Its evidence in patients with uncomplicated hypertension. *Arch Intern Med* 1984; 144:2171–2176.
25. Medical Research Council Working Party on Mild to Moderate Hypertension: Ventricular extrasystoles during thiazide treatment: Substudy of MRC Mild Hypertension Trial. *Br Med J* 1983; 2:1249–1253.
26. Papademetriou V, Price M, Notargiacomo A, et al: Effect of diuretic therapy on ventricular arrhythmias in hypertensive patients with or without left ventricular hypertrophy. *Am Heart J* 1985; 110:595–599.
27. Papademetriou V, Fletcher R, Khatri IM, et al: Diuretic-induced hypokalemia in uncomplicated systemic hypertension: Effect of plasma potassium correction on cardiac arrhythmias. *Am J Cardiol* 1983; 52:1017–1022.
28. Whelton PK: Diuretics and arrhythmias in the Medical Research Council Trial. *Drugs* 1984; 28(suppl 1):54–65.

HYPOKALEMIA AND INFARCTION
29. Nordrehaug JE, Lippe G: Hypokalaemia and ventricular fibrillation in acute myocardial infarction. *Br Heart J* 1983; 50:525–529.

30. Nordrehaug JE, Johannessen KA, Lippe G: Serum potassium concentration as a risk factor of ventricular arrhythmias early in acute myocardial infarction. *Circulation* 1985; 71:645–649.
31. Nordrehaug JE: Malignant arrhythmia in relation to serum potassium in acute myocardial infarction. *Am J Cardiol* 1985; 56:20D–23D.
32. Struthers AD, Whitesmith R, Reid JL: Prior thiazide diuretic treatment increases adrenaline-induced hypokalemia. *Lancet* 1983; 1358–1361.

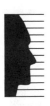
Affirmative Rebuttal
Kim Goldenberg, M.D.

Doctors Setaro, Black, and Moser appropriately suggest that there are a number of subcategories of hypertensive patients in whom potassium maintenance is likely to be beneficial. We agree that patients, with any degree of hypokalemia, who have underlying organic heart disease, and are taking digitalis preparations, or show high levels of ectopia are likely to be at increased risk for developing a fatal arrhythmia. Although Setaro et al. also recommend potassium maintenance therapy in diabetics, alcoholics, and those at increased risk for developing hepatic coma, they do not present data to support potassium maintenance in these patients. It seems somewhat capricious to allude to there being less than sufficient data for proving an increased mortality due to diuretic-induced hypokalemia and then not to present sufficient data to support almost half of one's recommendations.

Setaro et al. do appropriately present data from two large trials, the MRFIT and the HDFP. However, their presentation is somewhat flawed by mixing apples and oranges. For example, their Table 1 mixes coronary heart disease death rates from the MRFIT and total death rates from the HDFP. Although this admixture may be due to a problem in abstracting data from the literature, if coronary heart disease death rates were consistently shown from both studies (i.e., in patients with an abnormal ECG), the special care group from HDFP would show a higher, not lower as shown, mortality when compared with the referred care group. These additional data would further support the potential for diuretic- and possibly electrolyte-induced coronary death. In addition, their Table 1 refers to both studies as giving 5-year mortalities, when, in fact, the MRFIT was a 6-year study. The trends mentioned above, however, would remain the same.

Given the large sampling size in the MRFIT and the serious implications regarding diuretic-induced death, it is not surprising that the results of this trial have been carefully examined by a number of investigators. Setaro et al. point to Grimm (one of the MRFIT investigators), who suggests that the results could have occurred by chance. They also refer to a critical analysis of the MRFIT by Kuller (another investigator at an MRFIT coordinating center) but do not include Kuller's impression:

Thus, although the evidence is still incomplete, it is possible that the excess coronary heart disease mortality among MRFIT special intervention men with electrocardiographic abnormalities may have been caused by a combination of increased left ventricular mass in the presence of coronary atherosclerosis, and hypokalemia caused by good compliance with diuretic therapy and accentuated by stress-induced increases in circulating catecholamines.

Finally, Setaro et al. refer to the Glasgow High Blood Pressure Clinic in which the serum potassium level was the same for those who died of ischemic heart disease and those who survived: 3.71 vs. 3.72 mEq/L, respectively. It would seem more appropriate, however, to compare death and survivorship in a cohort of patients who are mildly hypokalemic, and who Setaro et al. suggest do not need potassium maintenance, than in normokalemic groups. Furthermore, although Setaro et al. recommend treating patients who become markedly hypokalemic (<3.2 mEq/L), we are not presented with any data to support this particular cutoff level and are not told if this potassium cutoff represents serum or plasma levels.

Whether a study indicates plasma or serum levels in its results may be important when attempting to determine a cutoff level for repleting potassium because the serum level may be higher, on the average, by about 0.2 mEq/L. This difference may determine whether patients in a study are designated as normokalemic rather than mildly hypokalemic. For example, Setaro et al. refer, in Table 3, to data from Papademetriou et al. to demonstrate that changes in plasma potassium level in patients with mild hypokalemia receiving hydrochlorothiazide do not significantly affect ectopia. However, plasma potassium levels of 3.3 and 3.4 mEq/L may represent serum levels of 3.5 and 3.6 mEq/L, respectively. Although a 0.2 mEq/L difference in potassium values may seem small, it represents the difference between normokalemia (serum potassium >3.5 mEq/L), mild hypokalemia (3.2 to 3.4 mEq/L), and severe hypokalemia (<3.2 mEq/L).

Setaro et al., at the conclusion of their position paper, mention both the safety and practicality of preferentially using combination diuretic–potassium-sparing agents instead of using thiazide diuretics plus potassium supplements. We completely agree with this concept. He also lists eight subcategories of hypertensive patients in whom potassium maintenance is important. It is not clear to me, however, what he means by potassium maintenance. It appears that recommendations for combination therapy are being suggested for seven of the eight subcategories, independent of the potassium level, as long as it is maintained at or above 3.2 mEq/L. However, an insulin-dependent diabetic (one of the subcategories) whose serum potassium level is at the upper limit of normal (4.8 mEq/L) would be at an increased risk of exacerbating any tendency toward hyperkalemia that might occur from an underlying hyporenin-hypoaldosterone state, even if followed up closely. Similarly, an elderly patient (another subcategory) with a high normal potassium level would be at an increased risk of hyperkalemia given the decreasing renin and aldosterone levels that occur with aging, as well as a decreasing glomerular filtration rate.

Admittedly, the decision to maintain serum potassium levels in the normal range is, in part, dependent on what one considers normal. For example, some laboratories designate a normal serum potassium level in the range of 3.7 to 5.1 mEq/L or higher based on their population distribution and assay technique. Although I wholeheartedly agree with Setaro et al. regarding the maintenance of potassium levels in patients who are severely hypokalemic, as well as regarding the mode of therapy, we disagree regarding the treatment of mild hypokalemia and relative decreases in potassium. I have purposefully not enumerated many subcategories for different treatment, as have Setaro et al., since the lack of correlation between blood and tissue potassium levels and the lack of specific data regarding risk-benefit analysis in many subcategories do not warrant it. Therefore, hypertensive patients receiving diuretics who also have other diseases that may predispose them to the development of hyperkalemia should preferably have their treatment individualized rather than subcategorized.

In conclusion, a number of large and small clinical trials suggest the need to treat mild hypokalemia, or any significant decrease in potassium level in hypertensive patients receiving diuretics, and to individualize potassium maintenance therapy when other disease states coexist. To let mild hypokalemia go untreated in hypertensive patients, many of whom are at unknown risk for myocardial infarction and sudden death, is to lose an opportunity for preventive intervention. Given the epidemic proportion of hypertensive patients in this country, a majority of whom are taking potassium-wasting diuretics, an ounce of prevention, by maintaining normokalemia, may well be worth more than a pound of cure.

Bibliography

1. Hyman D, Kaplan NM: The difference between serum and plasma potassium. *N Engl J Med* 1985; 313:642.

Rebuttal: Negative
John F. Setaro, M.D., Henry R. Black, M.D., and Marvin Moser, M.D.

In our original position paper, we sought to demonstrate that, though certain patients might benefit from routine potassium maintenance therapy, in general the case for a link between diuretic therapy, arrhythmias, and sudden death in hypertensives has been greatly overstated. Dr. Goldenberg in his statement correctly asserts that a patient with a serum potassium level of less than 3.5 mEq/L should be repleted. Yet we do not believe that an absolute fall of 0.5 mEq/L, for instance, from 4.5 to 4.0 mEq/L, merits treatment.

As for the large-scale multicenter clinical trials, evidence connecting diuretics with hypokalemia-mediated coronary deaths has not been convincing. The interpretation of MRFIT, quoted so frequently in attacks on thiazide treatment for hypertensives, suffers from several flaws. *Both* SI and UC groups received diuretics. No correlation could be demonstrated between mortality and diuretic dosage, nor did premortem serum potassium levels correlate with fatalities. In fact, higher mortality was observed in hydrochlorothiazide-treated patients *despite more pronounced hypokalemia* in those administered chlorthalidone. There was also a *lower* mortality in SI patients with abnormal baseline ECGs who received the higher doses of chlorthalidone. Last, UC group patients with abnormal ECGs had an unexpectedly *low* fatality rate, lower than UC patients with normal ECGs. Such results present insufficient evidence from which to draw major conclusions regarding antihypertensive therapy for millions of patients, especially when retrospective subgroup analyses have played such a principal role in the interpretation of these results.

As for smaller studies looking at diuretics, depressed serum potassium level, and ventricular ectopia, the 1981 work of Holland et al. may be critiqued in that it involved only highly selected cases with *severe* hypokalemia and no ectopia at baseline. As Dr. Goldenberg concedes, no increase in ventricular arrhythmias occurred in several other series, including those of Madias et al., Lief et al., and Papademetriou et al. despite hypokalemia in the 3.0 to 3.5 mEq/L range.

Only circumstantial evidence exists linking thiazides, hypokalemia, and arrhythmias in the setting of myocardial infarction. Though diuretics may cause hypokalemia, and there is an *association* between low serum potassium levels and malignant arrhythmias in the peri-infarction period, no causal effect has been shown.

Finally, much of the discussion of hypomagnesemia as it relates to heart rhythm disturbances is quite speculative. There is only the most tenuous connection between the successful use of intravenous magnesium preparations in the context of refractory ventricular arrhythmias and the possibility of arrhythmias being generated by thiazide-induced magnesium deficits in the hypertensive patient. Moreover, there is little hard justification for invoking hypomagnesemia to explain MRFIT or Medical Research Council results. Though the use of potassium-conserving diuretic agents may simultaneously reverse magnesium losses, it is not clear what the clinical import of such a maneuver would be.

We therefore stand by our initial conclusions: mild hypokalemia is well tolerated by the great majority of thiazide-treated patients, and most hypertensives do not need routine potassium maintenance therapy. The minority of patients who do require it are readily identified and treated and are probably most effectively treated with a potassium-sparing agent in combination with a thiazide diuretic.

Editor's Comments
H. Verdain Barnes, M.D.

One of the major current health thrusts in this country is controlling the blood pressure of an estimated 30 million hypertensives between the ages of 25 and 75 years. The most common form of therapy in use is an oral diuretic, of which a majority have potassium-wasting properties. The theoretic and known consequences of hypokalemia are common knowledge among physicians, but at what level of serum potassium these become clinically operative has been difficult to document. Therefore, when and how to treat those patients who do not have severe hypokalemia is still in dispute. Further complicating the issue is the lack of a strict correlation between serum and tissue levels of potassium and how to factor in the multiple variables that influence potassium homeostasis, such as insulin, catecholamines, diet, heart failure, and renal function, to name a few.

Since thiazide, a known potassium-wasting diuretic, is still considered by many to be the treatment of choice in a majority of mild to moderate hypertensives, it is of clinical importance to consider who should also be treated with potassium supplementation or a thiazide in combination with a potassium-sparing diuretic. The debate presented here addresses that issue. Four capable scholars submit their arguments: Drs. Setaro, Black, and Moser on the side of a more conservative and defined use and Dr. Goldenberg on the side of a more liberal use of potassium supplementation.

The positions taken on this complex issue are effectively presented, with all authors agreeing on some areas. First, they appear to consider the data on which to make a decision as not being as "hard" as they would like them to be. It is not surprising, then, that they do not agree on the interpretation of a substantial portion of the data presented to justify their respective positions. The rebuttal by Setaro et al. appropriately notes some of the problems that make the MRFIT data less than conclusive, but I agree with Dr. Goldenberg and his reference to Kuller that, although inconclusive, diuretic-induced hypokalemia may have been one of several potential contributing factors in the mortality observed in the study. Second, these debators agree that the studies of Madias et al., Lief et al., and Papademetriou et al. do not show an increase in arrhythmias in patients whose serum potassium levels ranged from 3.0 to 3.5 mEq/L. Third, they agree that the use of a thiazide plus a potassium-sparing diuretic rather than potassium supplementation appears to be a practical, safe, and effective approach to therapy. Finally, they agree about the necessity of raising the potassium level of those patients who are significantly hypokalemic (serum potassium < 3.5 mEq/L).

These authors vigorously disagree about the treatment of mildly hypokalemic patients as well as those with a relative decrease in their serum potassium level by more than 0.5 mEq/L below their individual pretreatment level. Relative or mild hypokalemia is a complex issue about which the literature is, in my judgment, incomplete, thus making it tenuous at best, if not impossible, to accurately assign a risk-benefit ratio. One must, therefore, decide whether he or she considers the literature to be suggestive enough of a potential cause and effect relationship between relative hypokalemia and "malignant" arrhythmias and/or sudden death. If the answer is affirmative, which I believe it is, then one only has to decide what level of hypokalemia to treat or prevent or to identify all the patient populations that are at the greatest risk of malignant arrhythmia, sudden death, or severe hypokalemia. Setaro et al. have expertly defined a formidable list of patient types (eight in number) that they consider to be at greatest risk. These are in general convincing, although a few would benefit by some supporting data, as Dr. Goldenberg has pointed out. In my view, if one includes the patients who fall into these eight categories, includes the estimated percentage of patients taking potassium-wasting diuretics who will develop some level of hypokalemia (i.e., up to 40% or 50%), includes the consideration that there is no effective method of predicting who will develop severe hypokalemia, includes the possibility that there may be an unidentified genetic component that permits or facilitates the development of severe hypokalemia, includes the increased risk of acute myocardial infarction in hypertensives and the possibility that hypokalemia may be one factor in the peri-infarction arrhythmia story (albeit not proved, as Setaro et al. point out), includes the potential role of magnesium deficiency in the hypokalemia story with thiazide diuretics,[1] plus the fact that malignant arrhythmias may be fatal and that sudden death is final, it seems clinically reasonable and perhaps vitally important to maintain serum potassium at or near a pretreatment level or at least well above 3.5 mEq/L in all hypertensive patients taking a thiazide diuretic. Therefore, the use of a combination thiazide and a potassium/magnesium-sparing diuretic or, if not tolerated, a thiazide alone plus potassium supplementation is clinically appropriate for virtually all hypertensives treated with thiazides.

This is true despite the fact that we are and should be trying to contain the cost of health care. Some will surely argue that such an approach is extravagant. On the other hand, I believe that such an approach would prove in final analysis to be cost-effective medicine in its truest sense.

Reference

1. Hollenberg NK, Hollifield JW (eds): Proceedings of a Symposuim. Potassium/ Magnesium Depletion: Is your patient at risk for sudden death? *Am J Med* 1987; 82(Suppl 3A).

High Calcium Intake Is Important in Preventing Osteoporosis in Women

Chapter Editor: H. Verdain Barnes, M.D.

Affirmative: Robert P. Heaney, M.D.
John A. Creighton University Professor,
Creighton University, Omaha, Nebraska

Negative: D.M. Hegsted, M.D.*
Professor of Nutrition Emeritus, Harvard
Schools of Public Health and Medicine, New
England Regional Primate Research Center,
Southborough, Massachusetts

*Supported in part by Grant RR00168 from the National Institutes of Health, Division of Research Resources.

Debates in Medicine 1:166–191, 1988
©1988, Year Book Medical Publishers, Inc.
0887-218X/88/01-166-191-$04.00

Affirmative
Robert P. Heaney, M.D.

A high calcium intake is both desirable and important for the American woman. The reasons are complex, but they begin with the fact that calcium is the principal cation of bone. Calcium must be present in the diet both to build a normal skeleton and to maintain adult bone mass in the face of obligatory excretory losses of calcium. Induced calcium deficiency in experimental animals regularly produces severe bone loss which is histologically indistinguishable from human osteoporosis. This bone loss is known to be parathyroid hormone dependent and can be prevented by prior parathyroidectomy, though at a cost of severe hypocalcemia. This phenomenon reflects the skeleton's role as a reservoir, used by the body to buffer changes in extracellular fluid calcium levels. Thus, there should be no question either that calcium deficiency produces osteoporosis or how it happens. But this is not the same thing as saying that all osteoporosis in all species is due to calcium deficiency; that would be quite wrong. We recognize the same situation with iron deficiency. It clearly produces anemia, but, of course, not all anemia is due to iron deficiency, nor can all anemia be prevented by high iron intakes.

Calcium, like iron, is a threshold nutrient. Below its level of dietary adequacy, bone mass varies directly with intake, whereas above the level of repletion—the intake threshold, as it were—further increases in intake produce no change in bone mass. What this means is that you can't make more bone just by ingesting more calcium, just as you can't make more hemoglobin just by ingesting more iron—you can't, that is, unless your intake is below the threshold of sufficiency. This intake threshold varies from species to species. It is high in the cat, and thus even brief periods of deprivation produce easily detectable bone loss. It is considerably lower in the rat, and one must combine low calcium intake with a significant calcium stress, such as pregnancy, before osteoporosis develops. The intake threshold for bone health in humans is the subject of considerable controversy.

Extensive studies both from England and from my own laboratory have shown a clear linear relationship between calcium intake and calcium balance. Low intakes are associated with negative balance and therefore bone loss; further, the degree of loss is related to the level of calcium intake. We find the same linear relationship if we evaluate balance as a function of absorbed calcium. Women with gross absorption of less than 300 mg/day are not able to sustain calcium equilibrium. Figure 1 presents true fractional absorption values in a large number of estrogen-deprived, early postmenopausal women, studied effectively at an intake of 800 mg/day—the current recommended dietary allowance (RDA). Nearly 80% of these

167

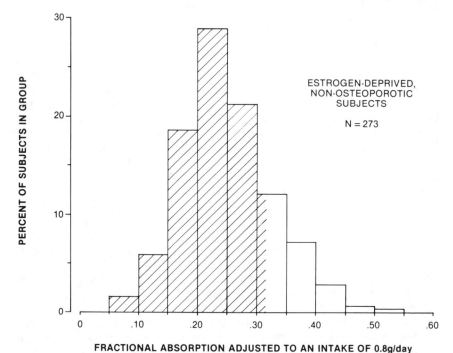

FIG 1.
Distribution of true fractional calcium absorption for healthy, estrogen-deprived, early postmenopausal women, adjusted to an intake of 800 mg/day. The cross-hatched bars represent the range in which absorption is insufficient to offset obligatory excretory losses.

women absorbed less than the amount required to offset obligatory excretory losses and were therefore in negative balance, i.e., were losing bone.

Obligatory losses in healthy U.S. women after menopause average about 180 mg/day. This figure is substantially higher than that found in women in nonindustrialized nations. This is one of the reasons why the calcium requirement for women of industrialized nations seems to be higher than for less technologically advanced peoples, and why fractional absorption must average at least 32% at an 800-mg intake. But, as Figure 1 shows, the majority of middle-aged women absorb less than that. (This poor absorptive performance could in theory be the result of bone loss, rather than its cause. Low absorption regularly accompanies primary bone wasting disorders. We do not believe that such is the case with most of these women, because their urine calcium was positively correlated with net absorption, whereas the opposite relationship is found in the primary bone wasting disorders.)

These findings suggest that the real intake threshold for most U.S. women is higher than their actual intakes. Consistent with this suggestion is the fact that recent analyses of the intake of contemporary hunter-gatherer peoples show that their average calcium intakes are in excess of 1,500 mg/day, or from two to four times the average intake in industrialized nations. Some anthropologists believe that the human genome is adapted to such calcium abundance, that a high intake is the "natural" intake for *Homo sapiens*. Thus, the much lower calcium intakes typical of western nations are, to that extent, a new environmental stress to which the species has not yet had time to adapt in ways that protect both calcium homeostasis and skeletal integrity.

That is the evolutionary challenge: to maintain homeostasis *and* to preserve the integrity of the skeleton. Calcium homeostasis has millennia of natural selection behind it. We recognize that the PTH–vitamin D hormonal system is the main component of that adaptive mechanism, and we understand in large measure how it works. What is unknown—and therefore the subject of controversy—is (1) just how low calcium intake in humans can drop (and for how long) without jeopardizing bone health; (2) what fraction of our population has impairment of this adaptive capacity; and (3) in those who do adapt adequately, what may be the long-term, nonosseous costs of chronically operating the adaptive mechanism at or close to its maximal capacity. The first two questions relate to bone health and disease (osteoporosis), and the third to the other calcium-related problems that have attracted attention recently (i.e., hypertension and colon cancer, among others).

Calcium Intake and Bone Health

Bone health in humans is a complex affair. During growth, bone mass is determined mainly by genetic forces. In the mature adult it depends more on mechanical loading and on normal gonadal and growth hormone status, as well as on nutrient intake. Menopausal women of industrialized nations are typically deficient in all three factors: low calcium intake, reduced physical activity, and, of course, estrogen deficiency. The relative importance of each for postmenopausal bone loss probably differs from country to country and from person to person and is still being worked out in general.

It is necessary to review the skeletal effect of estrogens before we can place calcium in the appropriate context. Women regularly lose bone when they go through menopause, and that loss can be prevented (or at least reduced to a male rate of age-related loss) by low-dosage estrogen treatment. The effect is confined to prevention of loss, and if estrogen therapy is started late, only stabilization of then-existing bone mass can be expected. The lost bone is not regained. This estrogen-related bone loss can be prevented only partially by high calcium intakes. Some of it, perhaps most, is estrogen specific.

Frank calcium deficiency is also prevalent at this time. Figure 2 shows the calcium intake data of U.S. women, taken from the National Health and Nutrition Examination Survey (NHANES II) study. Notice that the 25th percentile is at about 300 mg/day from age 20 onward. Even the median is at or below 500 mg by the time of menopause, and from age 12 onward, relatively few women get as much as the current RDA. Though the NHANES studies reflect intake at only a single time, the general experience of nutritionists is that women with low calcium intakes on a random day tend to have low intakes every day. In any case, as Figure 1 shows, even 800 mg is insufficient for most women. Clearly, women with even lower intakes must be losing bone.

Finally, inadequate mechanical stimulation is also part of the problem. Daily energy expenditure of typical sedentary women in their 50s has been shown in some studies to be as low as 1,100 kcal/day, or very close to the

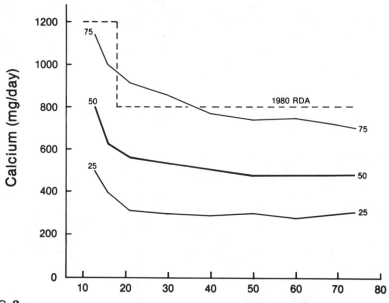

FIG 2.
Calcium intake data for U.S. women from the National Health and Nutrition Examination Survey (NHANES II; (1976–1980). The horizontal axis is age. The recommended dietary allowance (RDA) is indicated by the dashed line. The 25th, 50th, and 75th percentiles of actual intake at each age in years are shown.

level required to support basal metabolism. Mechanical loading of the skeletons of these women must be negligible. And yet mechanical loading is essential for maintenance of skeletal integrity, as has been shown over and over again in immobilization experiments. For example, up to 40% of the bone in the os calcis is lost in a period of bed rest lasting 24 to 30 weeks. (It is replaced when the subject resumes walking.) The importance of exercise is further emphasized by studies of total body composition, showing a nearly constant ratio of total body calcium to potassium in women as they age. This is despite loss of 30% to 40% of total body calcium over the postmenopausal period. This means that women lose muscle in the same proportion as bone. We in medicine have concentrated on the bones because they fracture, but it seems inescapable that much of the osteoporosis of the aging woman is not just a bone problem but a bone *and muscle* problem.

This interaction of hormones, nutrition, and mechanical loading in perimenopause explains a large part of the current controversy about the role of calcium and the frequent failure to find clear-cut effects in some studies. Though most epidemiologic studies have shown some relationship between current calcium intake and bone mass, in general the effect has been small, and to some observers it has seemed insignificant. For example, Garn analyzed data from the Ten State Nutrition Survey and found only very slightly more bone mass in the metacarpal in persons with the highest 15 percentiles of calcium intake than in individuals with the lowest 15 percentiles of intake. The differences, which were typical of many other studies, were simply not very impressive.

In some contrast are the now fairly familiar data from an eight-year-old study from Yugoslavia. Bone mass in the metacarpal was compared between groups living in two rural districts. One group had a relatively high calcium intake, the other, a low intake. Bone mass values at all ages were greater in the individuals with high calcium intakes. Of more importance, women with high calcium intakes had only one fourth the hip fracture rate of women with low intakes. There was, however, no difference in wrist fracture rate between the two districts. (This observation is consistent with the effects of intervention trials, which have generally shown no calcium effect on bone mass at the distal forearm, even when loss of shaft bone was completely prevented in the same subjects.) But there is another significant feature of this study. Both the high calcium and the low calcium individuals appeared to lose bone with age, and at about the same rate. Thus, though a high calcium intake may not be able to prevent age-related bone loss, it seems to assure instead the largest possible peak bone mass, achieved at about age 30 to 40. The study thus emphasizes the crucial importance of adequate intake during the years 12 to 35, when a strong genetic "push" to build bone still operates. Investigators in the United States have begun to look at this same question. Though it is difficult to do retrospective diet analyses, the few studies that have been reported all show that perimenopausal women who had high calcium intakes in early life have higher bone mass than women who had low intakes when young.

Several published intervention studies report small effects as well. Danish investigators, for example, have recently shown that, while a calcium supplement of 2.0 gm/day was able to retard the bone loss in shaft bone of postmenopausal women, it had no effect at all on the spine or on distal forearm metaphyseal bone, whereas estrogen completely prevented loss at all sites. Accordingly, these investigators concluded that calcium is not an effective substitute for estrogen. That conclusion seems hard to disagree with, at least as far as it goes. However, what is lost sight of in such experiments is that the subjects given estrogen were all estrogen deficient (i.e., they were all postmenopausal); hence, they all responded to estrogen. By contrast, most of the subjects given calcium could not in any sense have been considered calcium deficient. Hence, one would not have expected much of a response to calcium. Danish women in this age range average calcium intakes of 950 mg/day, nearly twice the U.S. average, and they have circulating vitamin D levels almost half again as high as U.S. women of the same age. Rather than conclude that calcium had no effect, I consider it quite remarkable that the calcium supplement produced any effect at all in such a population—one that, by most standards, would have to be considered relatively calcium replete.

Thus, the facts are not in dispute; it is their meaning that is controversial. I interpret these and similar studies to mean that calcium intake is limiting for only some middle-aged women. Others, for whom calcium intake is sufficient, predictably show no response. Mixing the two in any single treatment group inevitably dilutes the effect. Some women may even have calcium intakes that are low in an absolute sense but that are not the rate-limiting factors affecting bone mass in them (as, for example, would be the case with very sedentary women). One would expect no appreciable benefit from increasing the calcium intakes of such women.

Against this background we turn to the problem of osteoporosis. The only important feature of this disorder is bony fragility, and we now recognize that there are at least three classes of factors contributing to fracture. First is the injury itself and the propensity thereto; then the quality of the bony material, which we have recently come to understand includes both inappropriate architecture and inadequately repaired fatigue damage; and finally, reduced bone mass. Calcium intake is important only for bone mass. I make this point not to deemphasize the importance of either bone mass or calcium intake, but rather to place both in a larger context. All studies to date show clearly that reduced bone mass is an important risk factor, probably the single most important risk factor we recognize. In addition to its intrinsic fragility, low bone mass increases the amount of deformation of bone under load and so aggravates the tendency to fatigue failure; if one has ineffective bony architecture, reduced mass only compounds the problem. Therefore, low bone mass remains an important part of the osteoporosis problem, even though we now recognize that fracture is a more complex matter than we once thought. Finally, calcium intake is only one of the determinants of bone mass; inactivity, alcohol, smoking, drugs, and other disorders are also involved. In many women in our society today, calcium may not be the most severely limiting factor, even when it must be considered inadequate by other standards.

Thus, to grasp how calcium relates to osteoporosis, it is essential first to view osteoporosis as being a matter of bone fragility with consequent fracture, then to recognize that some, but not all, of that fragility is due to decreased bone mass, and finally to recognize that some, but not all, of that decreased bone mass is due to inadequate calcium intake. We have long since grown comfortable with this approach to an analogous disorder, anemia, in which not all of the problem is due to iron deficiency, and not even all of the iron deficiency is due to inadequate iron intake. Calcium remains important for preventing osteoporosis, just as iron is important for preventing anemia.

Disorders of Adaptation to a Low Calcium Intake

But what of the other side of calcium intake question, the costs of "successfully" adapting to low intakes? Abundant epidemiologic evidence from several populations now shows a link between low calcium intake and hypertension—a much clearer link, in fact, than can be found between most other nutrient levels and diet-related diseases. Several intervention studies show weak but clear blood pressure lowering from calcium supplements. The mechanisms responsible are now the subject of intense investigation, but many lines of evidence suggest a role for PTH and/or the vitamin D hormonal system. It is noteworthy in this regard that blacks, who have both lower average calcium intakes than whites and better calcium adaptive mechanisms, also have substantially more hypertension. Sustained high levels of one or both of the calciotropic hormones, made necessary if the individual is to adapt successfully to a low intake, are thought to alter intracellular calcium transport in susceptible individuals and thereby to increase the excitability of vascular smooth muscle.

Colon cancer presents yet another example of how low calcium intakes may aggravate a problem due primarily to some other cause. Mechanisms are uncertain, but recent studies show (1) that unabsorbed fatty acids and bile acids are irritating to colonic mucosa; (2) that a considerable load of these irritants regularly reaches the colon; and (3) that excess, unabsorbed calcium from the diet normally complexes with and thus neutralizes these irritants. Carcinogenesis in laboratory animals caused by colonic instillation of these irritants can be prevented by increased calcium intake. At low intakes in humans, there is little calcium available for this humble colonic function. Further, the more efficient the adaptive response to low intake, the more efficient the absorption and the less calcium will reach the colon. By contrast, at generous calcium intakes, absorption averages only 25% to 30% of intake, so there is ample calcium left over to bind unabsorbed irritant acids.

Summary

Osteoporosis, hypertension, and cancer are complex, multifactorial disorders. Calcium intake is only one of many factors involved. To deny that it has any role at all, simply because of the complexity of the issues, is to take refuge in a romantic world view where all things have simple causes. No one seriously maintains that every woman needs a high calcium intake, but clearly some women do. Undoubtedly some can adapt perfectly well to typical First World diets; some can do so even without paying the adaptive costs of increased risk of hypertension, cancer, and other disorders. But not all women get even minimally adequate intakes in the first place, and of those who do, not all can adapt. And not all who do adapt can do so with impunity. Since we don't know how to separate those who would benefit from a high calcium intake from those who would not, it is reasonable to assure a generous calcium intake *for all our population.* Thus, the recommendations of the National Institutes of Health (NIH) Consensus Conference on Osteoporosis (1984) continue to make good sense: that estrogen-replete middle-aged women should get 1,000 mg/day, and estrogen-deprived women, 1,500 mg/day.

The best way to achieve these goals is with foods. Ideally this would mean naturally calcium-rich foods. But except for dairy products, the calcium nutrient density of most of the foods readily available to American women is relatively low—lower than for most of the foods consumed by contemporary hunter-gatherer peoples. That fact, coupled with the low caloric expenditures of civilized peoples, is what is mainly responsible for the fall in modern calcium intake from higher primitive levels. So the next best thing is calcium enrichment of many different items in our food chain, thereby increasing their calcium nutrient density. This could range from staples (e.g., flour) to finished food products (e.g., orange juice). We have long since done the same thing for the problem of anemia by adding iron to white bread flour, and for the problem of goiter by adding iodine to table salt. Medicinal calcium supplements should be viewed as a last resort. Though it is better to get the calcium one needs from supplements than not at all, it is better still to get our nutrients out of the food chain rather than the drug chain.

Bibliography

CALCIUM NUTRITION—EVOLUTIONARY CONSIDERATIONS
 1. Eaton S, Boyd ES, Konner M: Paleolithic nutrition: A consideration of its nature and current implications. *N Engl J Med* 1985; 312:283–289.
CALCIUM AND OSTEOPOROSIS
 2. Heaney RP: Calcium, bone health, and osteoporosis, in Peck WA (ed): *Bone and Mineral Research*. New York, Elsevier North-Holland, 1986, vol 4, pp 255–301.
 3. Heaney RP, Gallagher JC, Johnston CC, et al: Calcium nutrition and bone health in the elderly. *Am J Clin Nutr* 1982; 36:986–1013.
 4. National Institutes of Health Consensus Conference on Osteoporosis. *JAMA* 1984; 252:799–802.
 5. Heaney RP, Recker RR, Saville PD: Menopausal changes in calcium balance performance. *J Lab Clin Med* 1978; 92:953–963.
 6. Horsman A, Marshall DH, Nordin BEC, et al: The relation between bone loss and calcium balance in women. *Clin Sci* 1980; 59:137–142.
 7. Matkovic V, Kostial K, Simonovic I, et al: Bone status and fracture rates in two regions of Yugoslavia. *Am J Clin Nutr* 1979; 32:540–549.
CALCIUM AND HYPERTENSION
 8. McCarron DA, Morris CD, Henry HJ, et al: Blood pressure and nutrient intake in the United States. *Science* 1984; 224:1392–1398.
 9. McCarron DA: Is calcium more important than sodium in the pathogenesis of essential hypertension? *Hypertension* 1985; 7:607–627.
CALCIUM AND CANCER
10. Lipkin M, Newmark H: Effect of added dietary calcium on colonic epithelial cell proliferation in subjects at high risk for familial colonic cancer. *N Engl J Med* 1985; 313:1381–1384.

Negative

D.M. Hegsted, M.D.

The recommendation that women consume 1,000 to 1,500 mg of calcium daily is, at the very best, unjustified by the available evidence. At the worst, it may be a disadvantage to those who follow the recommendation.

There is some evidence that high calcium intakes may slow the rate of bone loss in women with osteoporosis, but the combined therapy, including estrogen and fluoride with a high calcium intake, was much more effective. How effective estrogen and fluoride may be at more moderate calcium intakes is apparently not known. The main point to be made, however, is that many appropriate treatments for disease are not appropriate preventive measures and vice versa. Most drugs or surgical procedures do not indicate preventive measures; the removal of the carcinogens from the environment would not cure the carcinogen-caused cancer. Even if calcium slows down bone loss after osteoporosis develops, it does not follow automatically that it will prevent the disease.

The recommendation that women should consume such extraordinary levels of calcium is based on estimates of "requirements" obtained through calcium balance studies. By this technique one measures the intake and excretion (urine plus feces) of calcium and, by varying the intake, attempts to estimate the intake of calcium that will equal the urinary and fecal output. At this intake the calcium content of the body should be maintained. We concluded many years ago, however, that this method has no real validity. Milk and dairy products are not major items in the diet of most Peruvians, whose usual diet is relatively low in calcium. Using balance techniques, our Peruvian subjects had an average "requirement" of about 300 mg/day, whereas similar studies at that time, obtained primarily with U.S. and European subjects and summarized by Mitchell, indicated an average "requirement" of about 700 mg/day (Fig 3). Some have speculated that our prisoner subjects cheated and the calcium intake was actually higher than the analytical values for the diet. Whenever one deals with human subjects, this is always a possibility. These critics have not thought their criticism through, however. It is certain that if the calcium intake had been higher than our measured values, the excretion would have increased and more dietary calcium would have been required to achieve "balance." Thus, our estimates would have been too high rather than too low. Moreover, our results were not unique. Similar conclusions had been reached by others dealing with subjects accustomed to relatively low intakes.

In view of the difference in the results obtained with subjects of differing dietary backgrounds, our conclusion from these studies was that calcium balance trials tell us little, if anything, about physiologic requirements for

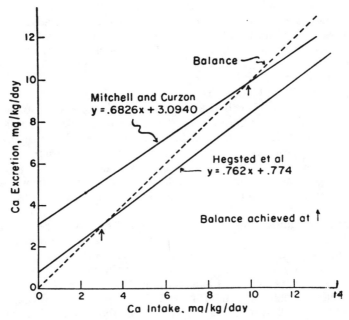

FIG 3.
Average calcium excretion observed in Peruvian subjects at different calcium intakes (Hegsted et al.) compared with the literature values compiled by Mitchell and Curzon obtained mostly with American and North European subjects. Calcium balance is achieved where the regression lines cross the line of equivalence (*dotted line*).

calcium, and that the apparent requirement is largely a reflection of the calcium content of the diet to which the subject is accustomed. Thus, it is not surprising that most studies in the United States, where dairy products are commonly used and calcium intakes are high by world standards, indicate a relatively high calcium need.

However, regardless of what one may think about such balance studies, it is certain that this general conclusion is true, i.e., that people adapt, within broad limits, to their usual calcium intake. If this were not true, most people around the world could not form and maintain their skeletons, and Americans and other milk drinkers would have extraordinarily large skeletons or be heavily calcified elsewhere. People who consume high-calcium diets must dispose of the calcium in some way, either by limiting absorption or increasing excretion. They are, inevitably, inefficient users of dietary calcium, whereas those living on lower calcium intakes are inevitably more efficient users of their dietary calcium. This cannot be denied. Calcium is an essential nutrient, of course, so calcium deficiency can be produced at some low level of intake. The question is how low this needs to be.

This is not the only problem with balance trials. The reliability of the data is rarely, if ever, known. Numerous studies show incredible apparent "retentions" of calcium and protein that cannot possibly occur. Calcium retentions in osteoporotic subjects, for example, have been reported that would obviously cure osteoporosis if they really occurred. There is no evidence that calcium will cure osteoporosis.

We and others could also easily show that, as expected, animals reared on low-calcium diets absorbed and retained their dietary calcium very efficiently, and their requirement, as determined by balance studies, was very low. Animals fed higher levels of calcium absorbed a smaller proportion of the dietary calcium and their apparent requirement was much higher. It is self-evident that if women, in general, required a gram or so of calcium per day, osteoporosis would be rampant in much of the world where calcium intakes are much lower than in the United States. Adaptation has to occur.

It is now well known that this ability to adapt to varying calcium intakes is largely, if not entirely, due to the vitamin D–derived hormone, calcitriol (1,25-dihydroxyvitamin D_3). Formation of calcitriol is increased by a low-calcium diet or by increased calcium needs, as in growth, pregnancy, and lactation, and decreased by a high-calcium diet or decreased needs, as in growth failure. Such a mechanism is obviously needed to protect against calcium toxic reaction, and the response in animals, at least, is extraordinarily rapid. Calcium intake or calcium need is probably not the only determinant of calcitriol level, but these kinds of protective mechanisms certainly explain, in large measure, why calcium deficiency is rare throughout the world in children and pregnant and lactating women when true calcium requirements are undoubtedly increased and calcium intakes are low by American standards.

The worrisome aspect of the recommendation that women should consume large amounts of calcium is obvious from Figure 4. These data on hip fractures were compiled from the literature by Gallagher et al.,[2] and the data on average calcium in the food supply are from the FAO (Food and Agriculture Organization) report. Although it is unfortunate that these data are so limited, they indicate that hip fractures become more prevalent as the calcium intake rises. Again, one may question any of the values in the graph; the data are relatively scant and their accuracy is unknown. It is known, however, that osteoporosis is an important health problem in Northern Europe and the United States, and that hip fractures are much less common in many parts of the world where dairy products are not commonly used and calcium intakes are relatively low. More epidemiologic data using improved methods to evaluate bone mineral content and calcitriol levels are greatly needed.

Since blacks are known to be less susceptible to osteoporosis, the epidemiologic data might represent variability in the susceptibility of ethnic groups. This seems unlikely, since there are many people of European

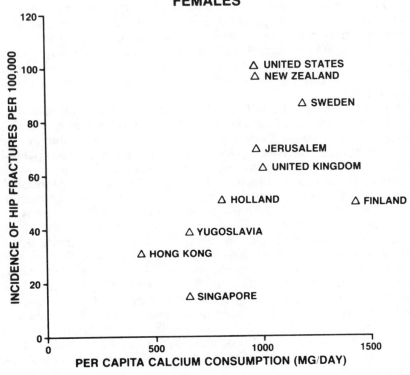

FIG 4.
Relationship between incidence of hip fractures in women in various countries (Gallagher et al.) and calcium available in the diet. (Data from Gallagher JC, Melton LJ, Riggs BL, et al: Epidemiology of fractures of the proximal femur in Rochester, Minnesota. *Clin Orthop* 1980; 150:163–171.)

extraction living in various parts of the world. Also, the similar question has been answered negatively for heart disease by the immigrant studies. These showed that acculturated immigrants develop the same disease pattern as the society they live in, and it seems clear that diet is the primary etiologic factor. Similar studies on osteoporosis in immigrants are urgently needed.

It has been adequately demonstrated that the absorption and utilization of dietary calcium are relatively poor in many, if not most, of the elderly women studied in the United States and Europe, particularly those with osteoporosis. Circulating calcitriol levels in osteoporotic subjects tend to be low, and calcium absorption can be increased by administration of calcitriol. Thus, the data are apparently consistent with the conclusion that for some reason or other, metabolic control of calcitriol levels is lost or becomes relatively inefficient. Apart from the therapeutic evidence, sex hormones and exercise appear to be clearly involved in protecting against bone loss. Whether they exert their effect via calcitriol appears not to have been studied.

Since the kidney appears to exercise primary control of circulating calcitriol levels, osteoporosis might be related to an abnormality in kidney function. In this regard it may be important to note (Fig 5) that the incidence of hip fractures is also positively related to protein consumption. In most but not all metabolic studies, a high protein intake increases calcium excretion. It is certain that high-protein diets place a substantial metabolic load on the kidneys, and there is at least the possibility that a lifetime on a high-protein diet might limit the capacity of the kidney to maintain normal control. Regardless of whether high-protein diets are involved in the genesis of osteoporosis, since more protein is likely to increase urinary calcium excretion, it would not seem logical to recommend that American women, who are already consuming diets with generous amounts of protein, should further increase their protein consumption. The average American woman is now presumably consuming about 500 to 600 mg of calcium per day. If they are to obtain nearly another gram daily from food, this would mean nearly another quart of milk daily. If protein intake is to be maintained near current levels, this would mean that they should substitute milk for meat. It is unlikely that this would be an acceptable recommendation.

Since it is obvious that animals and people (women at least until menopause) adapt to high calcium intakes by becoming inefficient users of dietary calcium, probably by continual depression of calcitriol levels, could this favor the development of osteoporosis? This is obviously unknown, but given the epidemiologic data, one can speculate that a lifetime diet that depresses calcitriol levels and induces inefficient utilization of calcium might undermine our capacity to adapt in old age when, for whatever reason, there is a tendency to lose bone.

The only preventive trial using calcium supplements that I am familiar with was completely negative but, also, did not indicate any detrimental effect of a high calcium intake. All preventive trials of the chronic diseases can be questioned, of course, since it might require 10 to 20 years or a lifetime before an effect can be seen. Nevertheless, this negative result combined with the epidemiologic data makes it highly unlikely that a high-calcium diet will prevent osteoporosis. Whether it will make the problem

INTERNATIONAL VARIATION IN PROTEIN AND HIP FRACTURES

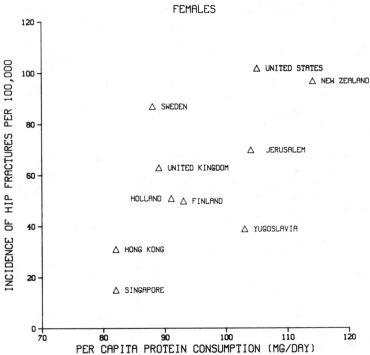

FIG 5.
Relationship between incidence of hip fractures in women in various countries and protein available in the diet. (Data from Gallagher JC, Melton LJ, Riggs BL, et al: Epidemiology of fractures of the proximal femur in Rochester, Minnesota. *Clin Orthop* 1980; 150:163–171.)

worse is problematic, but I consider it dangerous to ignore the epidemiologic data. Such data are, after all, the only measure of lifelong effects of the diet or other environmental variables that we have, and these cannot be assessed in controlled trials. Careful studies on immigrants would be helpful, but it must be remembered that dietary change in immigrants is slow. In some of the cancer studies, the change in incidence has only been seen in second-generation immigrants.

It is quite clear that we do not understand the etiology of osteoporosis, but it is of great interest to note that the epidemiologic data, limited though they are, suggest that osteoporosis, like coronary heart disease, many forms of cancer, diabetes, etc., appears to be largely a disease of affluent, western countries. This makes the diet a primary suspect, but it certainly does not suggest that it is the result of calcium deficiency.

It probably seems logical when people are losing body calcium to recommend higher intakes. However, this does not control bone loss, which occurs during bed rest or in weightlessness in astronauts, and has been questioned as possibly increasing the risk of kidney stones.

It may well be that surveys in the United States will demonstrate that osteoporosis is associated with low calcium intakes. Since small, sedentary women are known to be at increased risk and will have lower food intakes than large, active women, such data should be discounted unless these variables can be taken into consideration.

We customarily blame the food faddists and the unscrupulous for food fads, some of which are dangerous. This calcium fad, however, which has provided a bonanza for the pill industry, can be laid firmly at the door of the medical nutritionists and the dairy interests. There have always been "high calcium—dairy product—you never lose your need for milk" enthusiasts, but this recent round started with a report of a committee of the American Society of Clinical Nutrition, followed by the NIH Consensus Conference, and it would have been abetted by the Committee on Dietary Allowance of the Food and Nutrition Board if the National Academy of Sciences had not stopped the report.

In conclusion, calcium requirements assessed by balance trials will be high in people who customarily consume relatively high calcium diets or people who are losing body calcium. Unfortunately, the method simply doesn't tell us whether it is advantageous to be adapted to a high- or a low-calcium diet. Either is possible, but there is, as yet, no evidence that osteoporosis represents calcium deficiency; more importantly, the epidemiologic data on hip fractures raise the possibility that high calcium intakes may, in the long run, be detrimental. Metabolic studies, especially with subjects adapted to a high-calcium diet or osteoporotic patients, cannot answer the question.

A physician treating patients has to do whatever seems most appropriate at the time, and I see no reason why relatively generous intakes should not be used, although this does not appear to be a very effective approach. But in setting public health policy we should, first of all, be sure that we do not harm the population. The data on high-calcium diets and calcium supplements are not adequate to provide this assurance.

Bibliography

1. Christiansen C, Christiansen MS, McNair P, et al: Prevention of early postmenopausal bone loss: Controlled two-year study on 315 normal females. *Eur J Clin Invest* 1980; 10:273–280.
2. Gallagher JC, Melton LJ, Riggs BL, et al: Epidemiology of fractures of the proximal femur in Rochester, Minnesota. *Clin Orthop* 1980; 150:163–171.
3. Hegsted DM: Balance studies. *J Nutr* 1976; 106:307–311.

4. Hegsted DM, Moscoso I, Collazos C: A study of the minimum calcium requirement of adult men. *J Nutr* 1952; 46:181–201.
5. Riggs BL, Seeman E, Hodgson SF, et al: Effect of fluoride/calcium regimen on vertebral fracture occurrence in postmenopausal osteoporosis: Comparison with conventional therapy. *N Engl J Med* 1982; 306:446–450.

Rebuttal: Affirmative
Robert P. Heaney, M.D.

Dr. Hegsted is right when he stresses the difficulty of doing reliable calcium balance studies. (This is because of problems with accurate measurement of fecal calcium.) But he cannot have it both ways: he cannot reject as unreliable balance data supporting a high calcium requirement and then use his own balance data obtained from Peruvian prisoners to support a low requirement. Furthermore, his Peruvian studies are flawed in two crucial ways. First, even if they supported a low requirement, which I shall show is not the case, what does the calcium requirement of a Peruvian man who does not get osteoporosis tell us about the requirement of a North American woman who does? Next to nothing. Indeed, it might just be that the reason the Peruvian man does not get osteoporosis is precisely because his requirements are so low. Thus, such data beg the question. But there is an internal problem with the Peruvian prisoner study, as well. Dr. Hegsted and his colleagues used a low-residue diet, with calcium intake ascending from period to period, and they allowed only one day between intakes to clear the intestine of residue from the prior diet. Current data suggest that it commonly takes four days to accomplish this, or even longer. Thus, virtually all of the fecal excretion data from Dr. Hegsted's study are systematically underestimated. No wonder the requirement seemed low! Shift Dr. Hegsted's fecal data only two to three days to the left, and his study produces requirements very much like what everyone else has found.

So let us be clear. There are no calcium balance studies supporting a low calcium requirement, not even Dr. Hegsted's. The mean requirement Dr. Hegsted quotes from the Mitchell and Curzon review (700 mg) should not be confused with an RDA. An RDA is designed to be about 2 SDs *above* the mean requirement, and so the Mitchell and Curzon figure translates easily to an RDA of 1,000 mg/day or even higher. More to the point, all of the studies summarized by Mitchell and Curzon were performed in young adults; none was in women over 40, let alone after menopause, when it is well recognized that calcium utilization efficiency falls. Hence, the NIH Consensus Conference recommendations of 1,000 and 1,500 mg/day for middle-aged women (depending on estrogen status) still make good sense. Incidentally, Dr. Hegsted is right when he says that the 1985 RDA panel had raised the RDA (to 1,000 mg, in fact), and that the National Academy of Sciences had "stopped the report." But he is less than candid when he implies that it was the calcium recommendation that caused the report to be stopped. It was not. In fact, the calcium figure was considered conservative. It was the panel's recommendations on vitamins A and C that were controversial and that led to nonacceptance of the entire report.

Of course, none of the foregoing is to suggest—as I have stressed in my position statement—that a high calcium intake will prevent all osteoporosis. But increased intake *is* necessary to prevent the calcium-dependent cases and to assure that calcium deficiency will not be contributing to the cases of osteoporosis that are primarily due to other causes.

Dr. Hegsted states also that the typical Western diet is higher in calcium than the diet of most other cultures, largely because of the ingestion of dairy products after weaning. And yet we have a serious osteoporosis problem in the United States. So how could calcium have much to do with osteoporosis? I have stressed the importance of other factors, such as exercise, so I will not repeat that argument. But I must stress that, while it is true that First World citizens consume more dairy products than do persons from the Third World, the conclusion that adult calcium intake in other cultures is therefore low does not follow, nor is it supported by the facts. I have already alluded to the high calcium intake from vegetable sources alone (greater than 1,500 mg/day) that characterizes the diet of primitive hunter-gatherers. These are not exceptions. Coastal and riverine people have been found to have calcium intakes greater than 2,500 mg/day, derived largely from the bones of small fish, which are a staple in their diets. Vietnamese peasants, we have learned recently, soak bones in vinegar and drink the resulting liquid, particularly during pregnancy and lactation. (This potion contains roughly eight to ten times more calcium than a comparable volume of milk.) Central American Indians add lime to the cornmeal they use to make tortillas; Andes Indians add powdered limestone and a high-calcium ash to cereal gruels and other staple foods; betel nut quids contain added lime. More examples could be cited, but the point is that other cultures have low calcium intakes primarily when you base your calculation on Western food tables and food preparation practices.

Dr. Hegsted's comments on adaptation to high and low intakes are not really germane. In our own extensive work (200 normal middle-aged women) we have always performed our balance studies on intakes designed to match the woman's own self-selected intake, the one to which she is presumably adapted. What we found—and have published—was that women with low habitual intakes had not, in fact, been able to adapt; they were virtually always in negative balance. Only those with high habitual intakes were in calcium balance.

Finally, the suggestion that high calcium intakes might even lead to an increased risk of hip fracture is simply reckless. Dr. Hegsted's use of the Gallagher et al. data (see Fig 4) mixes ethnic and socioeconomic groups in an irresponsible manner. By contrast, whenever one works within the same socioethnic group, exactly the opposite effect is seen. The Yugoslav study to which I referred is a case in point: persons in the high calcium intake region had only one fourth the hip fracture rate of persons in the low intake region.

In most other respects I really find myself in substantial agreement with

Dr. Hegsted. High protein consumption does lead to increased calcium excretion and hence to increased calcium requirement, and that may be why the United States, with one of the highest standards of living in the world—and hence the ability to afford high protein intakes—has the highest hip fracture rate in the world.

I agree also that inadequate calcitriol production and/or responsiveness may explain in part the poor adaptation to low calcium intake that is so widespread among middle-aged and elderly women in Europe and in North America—why, in fact, Third World people may adapt better to low calcium intakes than we do. The reasons are not known, but several plausible causes have been identified. First is decreased solar exposure with age. Virtually all studies to date show falling levels of 25-hydroxyvitamin D (25[OH]D) with age. This is the principal storage form of vitamin D in the body. Furthermore, with age there is both a reduced capacity of the kidney to hydroxylate 25(OH)D to calcitriol, and a decrease in renal plasma flow and hence of delivery of 25(OH)D to the site where the hydroxylation occurs. Finally, some osteoporotic subjects have impaired intestinal mucosal response to calcitriol. Hence, for all these reasons, effective vitamin D status falls, and the adaptive response to low calcium intake becomes progressively more crippled with age.

However, it would be a mistake to attempt to solve this problem by widespread administration of calcitriol. This is a potent, dangerous hormone, and it should be used only under the most carefully controlled conditions. Rather, what must be done is to assure adequate, even youthful, levels of 25(OH)D in the plasma of middle-aged and elderly women. That means routine supplemental vitamin D intake of 400 to 800 IU/day.

Finally, neither Dr. Hegsted nor I can say with any certainty what the American woman will find acceptable. Dr. Hegsted suggests that an increase in calcium intake from food sources of 1.0 gm would require nearly an extra quart of milk, and that the American woman will not accept this. He is right, of course, about the calcium content of milk, but fluid milk is not the only, or even the main, alternative. Cheese and yogurt are excellent substitutes, and in fact, women do substitute them for meat right now. The amount of protein involved, even with a dairy food substitution, is only the equivalent of one Big Mac. So the change in eating habits required is not as impossible to achieve as Dr. Hegsted suggests. However, there are still other alternatives. There is the recent explosion of calcium-fortified foods (much to be preferred over pill supplements), such as calcium-enriched flour and calcium-fortified orange juice. There, for example, the choice would be not between milk and meat but between a low-calcium juice and a high-calcium juice, with the taste the same and no extra calories. In brief, it is well within our grasp to increase the average calcium intake of American women both safely and effectively.

Rebuttal: Negative
D.M. Hegsted, M.D.

The issue is whether or not there should be a national policy that advises all American women to consume very large amounts of calcium—1,000 to 1,500 mg/day—or raise intake to these levels by other means. Dr. Heaney prefers the increased consumption of dairy products, which are the only naturally available foods to achieve these ends, but has no objection to the fortification of foods or the promotion of supplements. As we have seen, this recommendation is being exploited by all interested groups: the dairy industry, the makers of pills and supplements, and now even the soft drink and cereal manufacturers. Dr. Heaney emphasizes the low calcium content of modern diets, but in fact the level of intake is relatively high compared with most of the world, and hip fractures, at least, are more common where the dairy industry is well developed and calcium intakes tend to be high. I find nothing in the argument to convince me that the health of Americans will be improved by such a policy, and until the epidemiologic data are explained, I feel we must entertain the possibility that such high intakes may be a health disadvantage.

The average American woman does apparently consume substantially less calcium than the RDA of 800 mg/day. Whether this should be a matter of concern is problematical. As I have indicated, this 800 mg/day value, like the recommendation for 1,000 to 1,500 mg/day, is based on balance trials and reflects a relatively high calcium intake in the subjects studied. It is noteworthy that other groups, like those that established the Recommended Intakes for the United Kingdom, recommend an intake of 500 mg/day. They quote Nordin as saying that osteoporosis develops in old people "regardless of diet" and conclude that it is apparently impossible to prevent osteoporosis with dietary calcium.

If American women do require two to three times as much calcium as women in most of the world, it is most unusual. I do not find any of the arguments valid, but if this is true we ought to know why. It would clearly imply that some factor other than calcium is of primary importance.

The issues of hypertension and cancer of the colon deserve a more extensive discussion. However, before we attribute the relatively low correlation coefficients between calcium intake and hypertension as causal, it should be noted that Garn's (personal communication) analysis of the NHANES data shows that hypertensive subjects are substantially heavier and fatter than nonhypertensive subjects, as would be expected, yet they either eat less or, more likely, report that they eat less—fewer calories, less calcium, less potassium, probably less of everything. Sodium intakes cannot be legitimately compared since the use of table salt was not reported. It is doubtful that either Heaney or McCarron will conclude that obesity or hypertension can be attributed to a lower energy intake or that we should recommend higher levels of food consumption to combat obesity or hypertension! Yet this is the reasoning in their evaluation of the calcium consumption data. Similarly, Feinstein finds that the standardized coefficient resulting from multiple regression analysis for diastolic blood pressure and body mass is .37, whereas that for calcium intake is −.04. Such a small coefficient becomes statistically significant when large numbers are involved. Others have also severely criticized McCarron's analysis. Pietinen et al. note that both calcium intakes and hypertension rates in Finland are among the highest in the world. Until the complex interrelationships between obesity, intakes of sodium and potassium, and many other things are better defined, attributing causal significance to small associations is very premature. Whether large doses of calcium have some pharmacologic effect on blood pressure apparently remains to be seen, but the Joint National Committee on Detection, Evaluation, and Treatment of High Blood Pressure does not find the calcium story credible.

Calcium may bind bile acids in the gut and increase fecal output. One hypothesis to explain the epidemiologic associations between diet and cancer of the colon is that the bile acids and sterols in the colon may be tumorigenic. However, the type and amount of dietary fat, which clearly have a major effect on sterol output and metabolism, are much more likely involved, and a role of fat is supported by the experimental animal and epidemiologic data. The probable protective effect of dietary fiber also has a much more solid base. Although I have not seen epidemiologic correlations between calcium consumption and cancer of the colon, it seems almost certain that these will be positive rather than negative.

Dr. Heaney argues that primitive people consumed levels of calcium in excess of 1,500 mg/day, and this is presumably the natural diet of man. This is similar to Linus Pauling's argument that our ancestors consumed large amounts of vitamin C and this should, therefore, be desirable. I find little reason to accept either estimate. Whatever the amount of calcium our early ancestors ate, it is more relevant to note that the majority of the world's population consumes even less calcium than most Americans, yet appears to be less susceptible to osteoporosis. Why?

Admittedly, it is quite unsatisfactory to say we simply do not know what level of dietary calcium should be recommended, but that is the current situation. Until we understand the etiology of osteoporosis, we have no justification for recommending major changes in the national diet, especially when such changes may not only be useless but possibly a detriment to health.

Bibliography

1. Committee on Diet, Nutrition, and Cancer: *Diet, Nutrition and Cancer.* Washington, DC, National Academy of Sciences, 1983.

2. Feinstein AR: Tempest in a p-pot. *Hypertension* 1985; 7:313–318.
3. MacGregor GA: Sodium is more important than calcium in essential hypertension. *Hypertension* 1985; 7:628–637.
4. Panel on Recommended Allowances of Nutrients: *Recommended Intakes of Nutrients for the United Kingdom,* Reports on Public Health and Medical Subjects No. 120. Department of Health and Social Security, 1969.
5. Pietinen P, Dougherty R, Mutanen M, et al: Dietary intervention study among 30 free-living families in Finland. *J Am Diet Assoc* 1984; 84:313–318.
6. Subcommitee on Nonpharmacologic Therapy, 1984 Joint National Committee on Detection, Evaluation, and Treatment of High Blood Pressure: US Dept of Health and Human Services publication 491–292:41147. National Heart, Lung, and Blood Institute, 1986.

Editor's Comments

H. Verdain Barnes, M.D.

Osteoporosis, a net loss of bone mass to a level less than that required for optimal mechanical support, is the most common metabolic bone disease. It is a feature of many inherited and noninherited disorders and is associated with others, ranging from osteogenesis imperfecta to hypogonadism to Menkes' syndrome. Most often, osteoporosis exists in the absence of other disease. The present debate focuses on its occurrence in postmenopausal women. At least two types of osteoporosis can be identified in this setting. Type I osteoporosis refers to a relatively small proportion of women who, in their early postmenopausal years to about age 65, have a relatively rapid and disproportionate loss of trabecular bone mass. Type II disease refers to the osteoporosis seen in women as well as men during and beyond their seventh decade of life in which there is a progressive loss of cortical as well as trabecular bone mass. Individuals with both types are at an increased risk of bone fractures (vertebrae and distal forearm in type I and femoral neck, pelvis, and proximal tibia and humerus in type II). Consequently, it is one of the most significant public health problems associated with aging. A recent estimate of the number of fractures in osteoporotic patients each year is close to 1 million, with a health care cost of about $1 billion just for their acute care. This frequency and cost along with the associated morbidity and mortality has generated a major research thrust in the area of epidemiology, etiology, prevention, and cure. Much has been learned about the epidemiology, and strides without definitive answers have been made in the other areas.

Our debators, Drs. Heaney and Hegsted, both recognized investigators in the field, have focused on the place of calcium in the broad area of prevention. Their excellent position statements and informative rebuttals state the crucial features of the current controversy regarding the potential efficacy of calcium in prevention. As I understand them, both agree that the precise etiology of osteoporosis is unknown and elusive, and that there is no known cure for these types of osteoporosis, as well there might not be, since there appears to be an inextricable relation to several inevitable components of the maturational aging process. Both agree that calcium is necessary for bone homeostasis and that calcium alone will not prevent osteoporosis or the associated bone fractures. They clearly disagree, however, as to what role a "high" level of calcium intake may play in conjunction with other potential preventive mesures.

It seems difficult to argue with Dr. Heaney's position that osteoporosis is a multifactorial disease, that calcium is at least one of the factors in some cases, and that for those women a high calcium intake is warranted. Unfortunately, as he states, "we don't know how to separate those who would benefit . . . from those who would not." A recent article by Abbasi and Hodgen,[1] suggesting that a short-term gonadotropin-releasing hormone antagonist test can identify those primates who will rapidly lose calcium after surgical menopause, may be a step in the right direction and probably merits study in women with surgical and naturally occurring menopause.

Although Drs. Heaney and Hegsted disagree as to the amount of calcium needed for bone homeostasis with aging, neither supports the wholesale use of calcium supplements currently rampant in the United States to the tune of a predicted $166 million in 1986.[2] Although Dr. Hegsted does not believe that a "generous" calcium intake is helpful, he sees "no reason why relatively generous intakes should not be used." Dr. Heaney, on the other hand, believes that a high calcium intake is beneficial to some, and since we don't know who, "it is reasonable to assure a generous calcium intake *for all our population.*"

From my perspective, the data available do not clearly define the physiologic calcium requirement at any age, do not support calcium intake as primary in the etiology of the majority of patients with type I or II disease, and are not convincing that a "high" calcium intake is preventive or curative. In addition, there are no prospective longitudinal data regarding the possible risks of long-term high ($\geq$1,500 mg/day) calcium intake. These questions all need to be answered, as well as, perhaps most importantly, who will benefit from a high intake. This will require innovative research and time. In the interim, I support an organized effort to educate our population about the body's normal need for calcium to maintain function and the importance of achieving a daily intake of between 800 and 1,000 mg, preferably by the use of natural or enriched foods.

References

1. Abbasi R, Hodgen GD: Predicting the predisposition to osteoporosis: Gonadotropin-releasing hormone antagonist for acute estrogen deficiency test. *JAMA* 1986; 255:1600–1604.
2. How important is dietary calcium in preventing osteoporosis? (Research News). *Science* 1986; 233:519–520.

Lymph Node Dissection Is Indicated in the Evaluation of Limited Malignant Melanoma

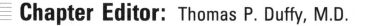

Chapter Editor: Thomas P. Duffy, M.D.

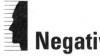

Affirmative: David A. August, M.D.
Assistant Professor, Department of Surgery,
Division of Surgical Oncology, Yale
University School of Medicine, New Haven,
Connecticut

Negative: Marc S. Ernstoff, M.D.
Assistant Professor of Medicine, Division of
Medical Oncology, Department of Medicine,
University of Pittsburgh School of Medicine;
Pittsburgh Cancer Institute, Pittsburgh,
Pennsylvania

Debates in Medicine 1:192–220, 1988
©1988, Year Book Medical Publishers, Inc.
0887-218X/88/01-192-220-$04.00

Linda Titus-Ernstoff
Department of Epidemiology, Graduate
School of Public Health, University of
Pittsburgh, Pittsburgh, Pennsylvania

Paul H. Duray, M.D.
Director, Division of Anatomic Pathology,
Fox Chase Cancer Center, Philadelphia,
Pennsylvania

John M. Kirkwood, M.D.
Chief, Section of Medical Oncology,
Department of Medicine, University of
Pittsburgh Cancer Institute, Pittsburgh,
Pennsylvania

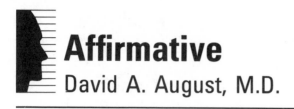

Affirmative
David A. August, M.D.

Cutaneous malignant melanoma accounts for just 1% of cancers and cancer deaths in the United States. Nevertheless, it plays a prominent role in many professional and public discussions of oncologic problems. In the past, melanoma has been thought of as a capricious neoplasm with an unpredictable course that may range from spontaneous regression or simple surgical cure to explosive dissemination and death. Recently, however, careful analysis of clinical and pathologic characteristics has yielded a more thorough understanding of the behavior of these tumors.

Despite intensive investigation of the use of chemotherapy, radiation therapy, and immunotherapy for the primary, adjuvant, or palliative treatment of melanoma, none of these modalities has demonstrated consistent efficacy. Surgery remains the only safe and effective method by which melanoma may be cured. Numerous studies have defined wide local excision (WLE) of the primary lesion with 3- to 5-cm radial margins and to the depth of the underlying fascia whenever possible as the best means of achieving local control. Although occasional patients may benefit from resection of distant metastatic disease, surgery usually has little to offer the patient with melanoma with tumor outside of the local site or regional lymphatics. In contrast to these well-defined surgical principles, the optimal treatment of the regional lymph node groups draining primary cutaneous melanomas is not widely agreed on. For decades, investigators have attempted to clarify the indications for lymph node dissection (LND) in the evaluation and treatment of limited malignant melanoma. I believe that recent data demonstrate benefit from a carefully planned and well-executed regional LND for most patients with melanoma. I shall support this contention by analyzing data that support the use of regional lymphadenectomy for many subsets of patients with malignant melanoma. Particular attention will be focused on the most controversial group of patients, those without clinical evidence of regional nodal or distant metastatic disease (clinical stage I). First, however, I will review some of the technical and surgical aspects of lymphadenectomy as they are relevant to the treatment of cutaneous malignant melanoma.

Technical and Surgical Aspects of Regional LND

Regional lymph nodes are the most frequent site of metastasis of malignant melanoma. In approximately 15% of patients, the regional lymph nodes represent the only site of metastatic disease at some time during the clinical course. Timely regional lymphadenectomy will cure these otherwise doomed patients. The presence of regional lymphatic metastases is of great prognostic significance, as patients with localized disease exhibit a 5-year survival of approximately 70% whereas those with regional disease have a 5-year survival of only 25%. Thus, regional lymphadenectomy is of great therapeutic and prognostic importance. Definition of the subgroups of patients who will gain most from the performance of this procedure requires an evaluation of its risks and benefits. The potential benefit of regional lymphadenectomy is different for each subset of patients and is addressed subsequently. At this point, a discussion of the nature of the procedure and the inherent risks will help to orient subsequent discussion. The surgical procedure required for removal of regional lymph nodes varies according to the location of the primary melanoma.

For patients with lesions of the head and neck, a neck dissection (sometimes including a superficial parotid dissection) is the appropriate procedure to be considered. Patients with truncal lesions may have metastases to either inguinal or axillary lymph nodes. These node groups also represent the regional lymphatic drainage for melanomas of the lower and upper extremities, respectively. Urist and coworkers reported the most extensive experience analyzing risk factors and surgical morbidity after regional lymphadenectomy for clinical stage I (local disease only) or clinical stage II (local disease and clinically suspicious regional adenopathy) melanoma in 204 patients. For those with head and neck melanomas, radical neck dissection was performed in 70% and modified neck dissection in the remainder (the latter procedure preserves the spinal accessory nerve and the sternocleiodomastoid muscle). In patients with trunk or extremity lesions, superficial inguinal or complete axillary dissections were performed. Short-term complications that extended the median hospital stay by 1 day were common and occurred in 21% of patients with neck dissections, 32% of patients with axillary dissections, and 29% of patients with inguinal dissections. With each type of LND, a chronic functional deficit occurred in roughly 8% of patients and chronic pain was a problem in 6%. Obesity and increasing age were associated with increased risk of developing a complication.

It may be asked whether less extensive regional LND procedures may be used to accomplish similar goals with less morbidity. The recent development of modified neck dissection procedures permits thorough sampling and removal of nodes at risk with less morbidity than that which accompanies radical neck dissection. These modified procedures result in fewer functional deficits and fewer problems with chronic postoperative pain. Urist et al. advocate the use of these limited neck procedures and report a corresponding decrease in morbidity. Unfortunately, limited axillary and inguinal procedures have no role in the evaluation and treatment of trunk or extremity melanomas. For patients with clinical stage I disease, it is imperative to perform complete lymphadenectomy so as to resect all potential disease-harboring nodes. In patients with clinically involved lymph nodes, at least two thirds have microscopic disease in adjacent clinically normal nodes. Resection of these nodes containing occult disease is required to achieve a cure.

When assessing regional lymphadenectomy for melanoma of the trunk, some clinicians are influenced by uncertainty regarding which lymph node group(s) are at risk. Despite anatomic guidelines such as Sappey's line, there are no reliable clinical predictors of which node basins are most likely to harbor occult metastases, and for some lesions axillary and inguinal node groups bilaterally may be at risk. However, recent experience with radionuclide cutaneous scans (especially technetium Tc 99m antimony sulfur colloid) shows these to be accurate and reproducible for determining the lymphatic drainage of truncal melanomas. They permit consideration of regional lymphadenectomy for a larger number of patients with melanoma.

Patients With Clinical Stage III Disease

Approximately 3% of patients with melanoma initially present with metastatic disease (clinical stage III). In these patients, regional lymphadenectomy is rarely indicated. In general, the survival of these patients will be determined by the behavior of their metastases, and LND is thus neither therapeutic nor prognostic. As median survival in patients with metastatic malignant melanoma is measured in months, it is rare that growth of involved regional nodes will cause local complications. Only if progressive nodal enlargement is anticipated to cause pain, functional disability, or skin breakdown with tumor fungation should regional lymphadenectomy be considered in these patients. Similar guidelines may be applied regarding the resection of any focus of metastatic disease in a patient with incurable melanoma.

Patients With Clinical Stage II Disease

For the roughly 15% of patients who present with melanoma limited to the primary tumor and clinically evident regional lymph node metastases, regional lymphadenectomy represents standard surgical therapy. The reasons for this are threefold.

1. Lymph node dissection can be of prognostic significance. Approximately 10% of patients with clinical stage II melanoma will be found to have pathologically negative nodes and thus have a prognosis much closer to that of patients with clinical stage I disease.

2. In a small but definite subgroup of patients with clinical stage II disease, tumor is confined to the primary lesion and the regional lymph nodes

(there are no occult distant metastases). With adequate excision of the primary lesion and thorough regional lymphadenectomy, these patients will be cured. Five-year survival is approximately 20% for patients with clinical and pathologic stage II melanoma in whom lymphadenectomy is performed. For these patients, regional lymphadenectomy is lifesaving. Until prognostic factors are defined that permit preoperative identification of those patients with clinical stage II disease not harboring occult distant metastases, it is justified to perform lymphadenectomy on all patients so as not to lose an opportunity for cure.

3. Unlike those patients presenting with distant disease, patients with clinical stage II melanoma can anticipate prolonged survival (median, 20 months). This time may allow significant growth of regional nodal metastases with resultant local problems from mass effect, skin breakdown, and ulceration. To prevent the occurrence of these disabling local complications, lymphadenectomy is indicated.

Patients With Clinical Stage I Disease

Controversy surrounding regional lymphadenectomy in patients with melanoma centers on the question of its timing in relation to resection of the primary lesion in those patients with clinical stage I disease. Some advocate immediate LND (ILND) to be performed at the time of definitive surgery for the primary lesion. Others argue for deferred LND (DLND) to be undertaken if and when patients on follow-up subsequent to primary resection develop signs suggestive of regional nodal involvement. Proponents of ILND note that approximately 20% of patients with normal regional lymph nodes on physical examination at the time of presentation in fact harbor microscopically detectable metastases. Regional lymphadenectomy will cure roughly half of these patients if it is undertaken before further tumor dissemination (the other half already have clinically undetectable distant micrometastatic disease that is destined to kill them independent of regional therapy). It is argued that delay in resection of regional lymph nodes containing micrometastatic disease may enhance opportunities for further tumor dissemination and thus eliminate the possibility of patient salvage through lymphadenectomy. Supporters of DLND note that by undertaking regional lymphadenectomy in all patients with clinical stage I disease, 80% are subjected to an unnecessary and possibly morbid operative procedure. Among the 20% who do harbor occult nodal metastases, it is suggested that delay of resection until such time as the nodal metastases are clinically evident does not increase the likelihood of distant dissemination. Both arguments hinge on the assessment of the risk of distant dissemination from occult nodal metastases left in situ vs. the risk of regional lymphadenectomy in patients without micrometastatic disease. Does delay in resection of micrometastases decrease the probability of cure in those

20% of patients with clinically undetectable nodal disease? What is the morbidity of regional lymphadenectomy in those patients not harboring metastatic disease? Clearly, if patients with micrometastatic disease could be identified preoperatively, few would argue against proceeding with ILND in these patients. Are there clinical or pathologic predictors of micrometastatic nodal disease in clinical stage I patients that would permit limitation of the use of regional lymphadenectomy to only those patients at high risk for pathologic nodal involvement?

Before addressing these broad issues, it is worthwhile to note two minor ancillary benefits of routine regional lymphadenectomy. First, the pathologic status of the regional lymph nodes is the most accurate predictive feature in patients with limited melanoma. Regional lymphadenectomy thus provides prognostic information that may be of importance to an individual patient. Second, pathologic staging of regional lymph nodes is a necessary part of any study investigating the clinical outcome of patients with melanoma. The staging information gained from a regional LND is critical to identifying and understanding the impact of experimental therapies.

The most important issue involving the controversy of ILND vs. DLND for patients with clinical stage I melanoma regards the effect of delay in the resection of regional lymph nodes harboring micrometastases on the probability of long-term survival. There are many retrospective and nonrandomized prospective studies published that argue either for or against ILND as a routine element of the treatment of patients with clinical stage I melanoma. Most of these studies indicate either no difference or an advantage in favor of ILND when 5-year survival is analyzed. This is despite a probable bias against ILND in many of these studies in that patients thought to have a poor prognosis may have been preferentially chosen for this more extensive therapy. Though suggestive, these data are at best difficult to interpret. Analysis of these studies is also confounded because the majority of patients subjected to ILND do not have micrometastases and the majority of patients not undergoing ILND are also free of occult nodal disease. These two groups of patients would be expected to have similar survival independent of the type of regional nodal therapy offered. Thus, these patients may mask any beneficial effect of ILND in node-positive patients. If one analyzes these retrospective and nonrandomized prospective studies so as to compare only patients with nodal disease at the time of ILND with those who develop clinically evident nodal disease subsequent to WLE alone, the data become more suggestive. They demonstrate a trend toward improved survival attributable to ILND. This advantage may range from nil to as high as 30% at 5 years.

Two prospective randomized trials have been conducted to better address the controversy of ILND vs. DLND in the treatment of clinical stage I melanoma. It is data from these trials that are most widely quoted against the use of ILND. The larger of the two trials is a WHO multicenter international study of 553 patients with melanoma of the upper and lower extremities. This study accrued patients in the period 1967 to 1974. Patients were randomized to receive WLE and ILND or WLE alone. In the first 5 years after treatment, patients randomized to receive ILND were followed up quarterly. In this same period, follow-up was carried out monthly in patients randomized to receive WLE only. From the sixth year on, both groups were followed up at 6-month intervals. By actuarial analysis, approximately 75% of patients in both groups were alive at 5 years and 60% at 10 years from the time of diagnosis. Analysis of the two treatment groups indicates that they were balanced for a variety of possibly prognostic features. No significant difference in 5- or 10-year survival was seen in subsets defined by sex, age, maximum lesion diameter, lesion thickness, or level of invasion. These subsets were analyzed retrospectively and were not stratified prospectively. Comparison of the 54 patients found to have micrometastatic disease at the time of ILND with the 64 who developed regional lymph node metastases and underwent DLND during subsequent follow-up showed a 50% vs. 44% survival at 5 years and 35% vs. 23% survival at 10 years, both favoring ILND. There was no statistical significance to these differences, possibly because of the small numbers of patients.

The second prospective randomized study addressing this issue was conducted by the Mayo Clinic, Rochester, Minn. In the period 1972 to 1977, the investigators randomized 171 patients with clinical stage I melanoma within a three-arm study. Sixty-two patients underwent DLND only if clinically warranted, 54 patients had ILND, and 55 patients had planned regional lymphadenectomy performed 3 months after resection of the primary lesion. Comparison of the three groups revealed them to be balanced for all known prognostic features. Overall, there were no significant differences in survival or disease-free survival between the three groups at 5 or 10 years following initial resection. No subset analysis was performed to determine whether any particular group of patients might have benefitted from ILND. Among those patients randomized to receive DLND, 26% (16/62) had a "melanoma-related event" (local, regional, or distant recurrence) following primary resection. In the ILND group and the group undergoing planned node dissection at 3 months, there was a 16% (17/109) incidence of melanoma-related events. This difference was statistically significant. Only 18 of the patients in the DLND group ultimately developed regional nodal metastases and only seven patients in the other groups had positive LNDs. Because of the small numbers, no comparison could be made between these patients of greatest interest.

These two prospective, randomized studies invalidate the concept of *indiscriminate* ILND for *all* patients with clinical stage I melanoma. When examined carefully, however, neither study offers persuasive evidence against the use of ILND in most patients with clinical stage I melanoma. The WHO study enlisted only patients with extremity tumors (roughly 50%

of all patients). These in general are lesions with better prognosis. Over 80% of the patients in this study were female, and this too is associated with a better prognosis. As patients with thin primary lesions are at minimal risk for either regional or distant spread, and patients with thick primary lesions are likely to have occult distant disease, maximum benefit from ILND would be expected to accrue to those patients with primary lesions of intermediate Breslow thickness. Of the 338 patients in the study in whom tumor thickness could be evaluated, only 206 (61%) had intermediate lesions 1 to 3.9 mm thick. Thus, by virtue of tumor location, sex, and tumor thickness, the patients in the WHO study are among those least likely to benefit from ILND. Nevertheless, in the subgroup of greatest interest, those found to have regional lymph node metastases at the time of ILND or subsequently, there was indeed a suggestion of improved long-term survival in those randomized to receive ILND. Although the WHO study utilized extensive retrospective subgroup analysis, there was no pre-randomization stratification of patients according to prognostic features such as lesion thickness or depth of invasion. Without prospective stratification, subgroup analysis to define patients who might benefit from ILND is inconclusive. The authors also note that DLND is warranted only if close follow-up is achievable. Although the Mayo Clinic protocol included some patients with truncal lesions (20% of all patients), similar criticisms may be directed at this study. Though the study failed to demonstrate a survival benefit from ILND, there was a clear reduction in tumor-related events in patients in the ILND group.

A number of prospective studies support the use of ILND in large subgroups of patients with clinical stage I disease. Among the clinicopathologic features that have been associated with poor outcome in patients with melanoma are increasing thickness of the primary tumor, depth of invasion (Clark's level), superficial spreading or nodular histology, location of the primary on the trunk or head and neck, increasing diameter of the primary, ulceration of the primary, the presence of microscopic or gross satellite lesions, and the presence and extent of regional lymph node involvement. It is these clinicopathologic features that may define subsets of patients who will benefit from routine ILND.

Urist and coworkers retrospectively analyzed data collected prospectively on 453 patients with superficial spreading or nodular melanoma. A multifactorial analysis was conducted evaluating a variety of clinical and pathologic factors to determine their prognostic value. Patients undergoing ILND had a statistically significant survival advantage over patients initially undergoing WLE alone for melanomas with a Breslow thickness of 1.5 to 3.99 mm. This survival advantage was not statistically evident for melanomas less than 1.5 mm or greater than 3.99 mm in thickness. McCarthy and coworkers analyzed data collected prospectively on 2,347 patients with clinical stage I melanoma of the extremities or trunk with a superficial spreading or nodular histology. In roughly three quarters of these patients, the initial therapy consisted of WLE alone; the remainder underwent WLE and ILND. Men with lesions of intermediate thickness (1.6 to 3 mm) benefited most from ILND when 10-year survival rates were analyzed. This was true for lesions of the trunk and of the extremities. Though women with truncal lesions did not appear to benefit from ILND, those with extremity lesions of intermediate thickness had statistically significant improvement in 10-year survival. Balch et al. retrospectively analyzed 156 patients with clinical stage I melanoma with head and neck, trunk, or extremity lesions with regard to the effect of their initial surgical treatment on actuarial 5-year survival. Patients with lesions thinner than 0.77 mm had a zero incidence of nodal metastases, those with lesions 0.77 to 1.49 mm had a 25% incidence of regional metastases, and those with lesions 1.5 mm or greater had over a 50% incidence of regional node metastases. A statistically significant increase in survival was found for those patients whose lesions were from 0.77 to 3.99 mm thick who underwent ILND vs. DLND.

Although these three studies were not randomized, they strongly suggest that there are subgroups of patients with clinical stage I melanoma whose long-term survival is improved if their initial surgical therapy includes regional lymphadenectomy. This survival advantage is most likely to be observed in those patients with either superficial spreading or nodular histologies and with intermediate Breslow thickness (0.77 or 1.50 to 4 mm). Patients with head and neck primaries and possibly truncal primaries might also benefit from ILND.

Overview

The preceding analyses, rather than unambiguously defining the role of LND in the evaluation of limited malignant melanoma, highlight continuing uncertainty regarding the most appropriate use of regional lymphadenectomy. Nevertheless, a number of definitive statements can be made. The appropriate procedures can be performed with acceptable morbidity (<10%) and no mortality. Regional lymphadenectomy, by defining the pathologic status of the draining nodal basins, is the most accurate predictor of long-term survival. If prognostic information is important (as in research protocols), adenectomy is indicated. In approximately 15% of patients with malignant melanoma, the regional lymph nodes will at some time represent the only site of metastatic disease, and in these patients, regional lymphadenectomy is curative. For the 15% of patients who present with clinical stage II disease, ILND is almost always indicated, and for 20% of these patients it will be lifesaving. Of the 85% of patients with melanoma who initially present with clinical stage I disease, roughly 60% (approximately 50% of all patients with melanoma) will have primary tumors of intermediate thickness (0.77 to 3.99 mm). This group of patients may potentially derive the greatest survival benefit from ILND. Other patients with poor prognostic features such as tumor ulceration, anatomic location on head and neck or trunk, and men may also derive significant benefit from ILND. These patients make up well over half of all patients with melanoma and thus support the contention that LND is indicated in the evaluation of most limited melanomas. Clearly, it is only through large, prospective, randomized trials that stratify patients according to prognostic features that the optimal role for regional lymphadenectomy in the treatment of limited malignant melanoma can be defined.

Bibliography

1. Balch CN: Clinical management of cutaneous melanoma, in McKenna RJ, Murphy GT (eds): *Fundamentals of Surgical Oncology*. New York, Macmillan Publishing Co, 1986, pp 420–439.
2. Mastrangelo MJ, Baker AR, Katz HR: Cutaneous melanoma, in DeVita VT, Hellman S, Rosenberg SA (eds): *Principles and Practice of Oncology*, ed 2. Philadelphia, JB Lippincott Co, 1985, pp 1371–1422.
3. Sim FH, Taylor WF, Pritchard DJ, et al: Lymphadenectomy in the management of stage I malignant melanoma: A prospective randomized study. *Mayo Clin Proc* 1986; 61:697–705.
4. Veronesi U, Adamus J, Bandiera DC, et al: Delayed regional lymph node dissection in stage I melanoma of the skin of the lower extremities. *Cancer* 1982; 49:2420–2430.
5. Urist MM, Maddox WA, Kennedy JE, et al: Patient risk factors and surgical morbidity after regional lymphadenectomy in 204 melanoma patients. *Cancer* 1983; 51:2152–2156.
6. Balch CN, Murad TN, Soong S-J, et al: Tumor thickness as a guide to surgical management of clinical stage I melanoma patients. *Cancer* 1979; 43:883–888.
7. McCarthy WH, Shaw HM, Milton GW: Efficacy of elective lymph node dissection in 2347 patients with clinical stage I malignant melanoma. *Surg Gynecol Obstet* 1985; 161:575–580.
8. Urist MM, Balch CN, Soong S-J, et al: Head and neck melanoma in 534 clinical stage I patients: A prognostic factors analysis and results of surgical treatment. *Ann Surg* 1984; 200:769–775.

Negative

Marc S. Ernstoff, M.D., Linda Titus-Ernstoff, Paul H. Duray, M.D., and John M. Kirkwood, M.D.

Although Hippocrates was the first to describe pigmented skin tumors, the earliest use of the term melanoma is attributed to Carswell in 1836.[1] Pemberton introduced lymph node dissection (LND) as an adjunct to local excision in the surgical treatment of this disease in 1858.[1] Handley[2] reported pathologic evidence of lymph node metastases in 1907 and advocated LND as a method of controlling the spread of occult regional disease. Although Handley's conclusions were based on a single autopsy, LND was quickly adopted as standard therapy for melanoma. The procedure gained further support from Stewart et al.,[3] who reported survival benefit among patients undergoing LND in 1932, and from Pack et al.,[4] who reported occult metastases in 42% of regional lymph node specimens in 1945.

To date, excision of the primary tumor provides the only means to prevent recurrence of melanoma. The lack of effective treatment for regional and distant metastatic melanoma underscores the importance of early and complete surgical excision of localized tumor.[5, 6] Dissection of the regional draining lymph nodes has been advocated both to remove regional disease and to prevent distant dissemination.[7–14]

It is generally agreed that LND offers no potential therapeutic benefit for shallow, low-risk primary melanoma (Clark level I and II or Breslow depth <0.76 mm) or very deep lesions at highest risk of distant metastases (Clark level V or Breslow depth >3.99 mm). However, the role of LND in the treatment and evaluation of clinical stage I melanoma of intermediate depth is a subject of continuing debate.[8–10, 15–19] Resolution of this controversy requires a determination of the true benefits and risks associated with LND. Major issues for consideration can be summarized by the following questions:

1. Does prophylactic LND improve survival among patients with clinical stage I cutaneous melanoma?

2. Does prophylactic LND control regional disease?

3. Does prophylactic LND contribute to the identification of individuals at high risk for metastases who might subsequently benefit from adjuvant therapy?

4. Does prophylactic LND provide tumor that may be utilized for immunization programs of potential utility to the host?

5. What is the morbidity associated with prophylactic LND?

The majority of published reports dealing with the usefulness of LND in the evaluation and treatment of melanoma are based on retrospective or nonrandomized prospective studies.[9-13, 15, 18, 20-23] The influence of LND on survival has also been assessed in two randomized prospective studies,[16, 17, 24] both of which report a lack of significant survival advantage among recipients of prophylactic LND. The recently published literature will be reviewed to clarify the utility of prophylactic LND in the context of the above questions.

Microstaging, LND, and Prognosis

Microstaging of tumors was introduced in 1969 by Clark et al.[25] and independently by Breslow[26] in 1970. Clark's method of microstaging is based on the measure of tumor invasion through the layers of the skin. Breslow's method measures the actual depth of the tumor, in millimeters, from the top of the granular cell layer of the skin. Although there are many other prognostic factors, including gender of the patient, site, ulceration, growth patterns, and diameter of the lesion, microstaging has most consistently demonstrated its value as a predictor of regional lymph node metastases and survival outcome.*

Despite the prognostic value of standardized microstaging techniques, it is difficult to identify patients with clinical stage I disease who have subclinical lymph node metastases.[8, 12, 27, 30] The difficulty of predicting the existence of microscopic regional lymphatic involvement appears to support the utility of routine LND for patients with clinical stage I melanoma. However, even if one assumes a survival benefit of prophylactic removal of occult regional metastases, only a fraction of all patients with clinical stage I disease are eligible for such benefit. Among patients with very shallow lesions (<0.76 mm), risk for regional or distant metastases is low. Among patients with deeper lesions, a certain proportion will develop distant metastases without ever manifesting evidence of regional involvement. Data from several studies suggest that between 15% and 35% of patients with clinical stage I disease will eventually relapse without evidence of prior lymph node metastases.[10, 11, 13, 16, 17] Data from the WHO Melanoma Group Register show that approximately 56% of patients with clinical stage I disease treated with wide local excision (WLE) remained disease free at 10-year follow-up. Among the 44% of patients with WLE whose disease recurred during the same period, about half recurred first in the regional lymph nodes, 31% relapsed simultaneously at regional and distant sites, and 22% relapsed at distant sites only. These data clearly indicate that the dissemination of metastatic disease to distant sites is not always associated with clinically manifest regional lymph node disease. In fact, only half of the patients who relapsed were eligible for potential benefit due to prophy-

*References 8–11, 13–15, 18, 20, 22, 27–29.

lactic LND. More to the point, of the entire series of patients with clinical stage I melanoma in the WHO Register, only 21% were eligible for such benefit. The focus of interest is whether the fraction of patients who will relapse first at regional lymph nodes can indeed benefit from prophylactic dissection.

Table 1 summarizes the results of eight nonrandomized studies. Two retrospective studies provide statistical evidence of survival benefit associated with LND in a subgroup of patients with clinical stage I disease.[9, 15] Balch et al.[15] demonstrate improvement in survival associated with LND among patients with primary tumors ranging in depth from 0.76 to 3.99 mm, with particular benefit to patients with tumor depth of 1.5 to 3.99 mm. Breslow[9] reports survival benefit with LND for patients with tumors exceeding 1.5 mm in depth. In addition, a nonrandomized prospective study reports survival advantage for clinical stage I melanoma when tumor depth exceeds Clark level II.[10] Although the data for this study were collected prospectively, lack of randomization of patients to treatment protocols introduces many of the potential biases inherent in retrospective studies.

Several investigators report survival advantage due to elective LND despite equivocal statistical results. Kapelanski et al.[13] found a slight but statistically nonsignificant improvement in 5-year survival for patients with clinical stage I melanoma with prophylactic LND. The data of Wanebo et al.[14] show an association between prophylactic LND and 5-year survival

TABLE 1.
Eight Randomized Studies of LND

Source	No.	WLE	WLE + LND	5-yr Disease-Free Survival, No. (%)	
				WLE	WLE + ELND*
Fortner et al.[11]	404	145	259	102 (70)	197 (76)
Kapelanski et al.[13]	91	65	26	36 (55)	17 (65)
Balch et al.[21]	320	156	164	98 (63)	139 (85)
Bagley et al.[22]	103	59	44	50 (85)	32 (73)
McCarthy et al.[23]	207	162	45	131 (81)	33 (73)
Blois et al.[18]	222	111	111	83 (75)	85 (77)
Wanebo et al.[14]	151	38	113	27 (71)	92 (81)
Breslow[9]	138	96	42	67 (70	31 (74
Total	1,636	832	804	594 (71)	626 (78)

*ELND indicates elective LND.

among patients with Clark level III tumors; however, this difference in survival for the two surgical treatment groups was not evident after 9 years of follow-up. In a large retrospective series, Milton et al.[20] found evidence of improved survival associated with prophylactic LND among men with axial tumors of intermediate thickness. Among women, survival benefit with LND was noted for those with axial and extremity tumors of intermediate thickness and extremity tumors greater than 3.0 mm in depth. However, the survival differences reported in this study were not statistically significant. Fortner et al.[11] retrospectively evaluated survival outcome for three treatment groups: WLE only, WLE plus prophylactic LND, and WLE plus therapeutic LND. Although similar survival rates were noted for the three groups, the investigators conclude that the presence of metastases in the pathology of dissected nodes provides sufficient rationale for the use of prophylactic LND.

Two nonrandomized studies report no survival benefit among patients following prophylactic LND. The retrospective study by Bagley et al.[22] of survival and prophylactic LND used Breslow depth in conjunction with the Clark level to divide patients into categories of low, moderate, and high risk. In this study, no survival benefit was noted for patients with prophylactic LND. Blois et al.[18] conducted a nonrandomized prospective study in which 222 patients with melanoma, half with LND and half without, were selected to create 111 dichotomous pairs. Individual members of each pair were matched for level of tumor, site of primary, and gender. Study results showed no difference in survival between the two surgical treatment groups.

The limitations of retrospective studies and the sources of bias that may influence the results of these studies are widely recognized by epidemiologists.[32–34] In the context of understanding the relationship between prophylactic LND and survival, the direction of operating biases depends on the interrelationships of (1) the disease characteristics of a particular sample of melanoma cases, including prevalence of occult regional metastases, metastatic potential, and the proportion of advancing disease mediated by the lymphatics; and (2) medical care variables, including systematic selection of candidates for LND according to subtle differences in staging and the timing of LND intervention. Inconsistencies in the results of various nonrandomized studies evaluating the effect of elective LND on survival may reflect differences in the interplay of these factors across study populations.

Balch et al.[15] have compiled a large series of patients with clinical stage I melanoma that provides persuasive and recent support for survival benefit due to LND. In this study, cases with clinical stage I melanoma identified by tumor registries at the University of Alabama and in New South Wales, Australia, were compared for surgical treatment and survival outcome. Although the methodology of this study is described as predominately prospective (and tumor registry data were for the most part collected prospectively), the investigation itself appears to follow a retrospective design: the relationship between LND and survival was evaluated among incident cases of melanoma already identified by the registries.

The lack of randomization in this study introduces potential bias resulting from the influence of factors that determine choice of surgical treatment. Selection bias, operative when patients with LND differ systematically from those whose nodes are not dissected, can affect availability of follow-up information and distort study results. There are various ways in which selection bias can be introduced to nonrandomized studies. If a subset of patients selected for WLE is subjectively but correctly identified for favorable outcome, requires little medical surveillance, and is more likely to relocate geographically than WLE patients who relapse, then survival information for the healthy subset may not be available to the tumor registry. Because of loss to follow-up, this subset of healthy WLE patients will be excluded from the study. If loss to follow-up occurs most frequently among the subset of healthy WLE patients, then the initial selection bias results in an artifactual survival benefit for patients with LND.

A form of self-selection bias may result in lower frequency of occult regional metastases and extended survival among patients treated with prophylactic LND. Patient or physician attitudes toward health care may result in earlier diagnosis with clinically undetectable survival advantage and influence the decision favoring aggressive surgical treatment. In this setting, health care attitudes and behaviors act as a confounder in the relationship between surgical treatment and survival.

In addition to generic limitations inherent in retrospective methodology, the graphic presentation of these study results may exaggerate the relationship between LND and survival. Actuarial curves for the two surgical treatment groups appear to be extrapolated beyond available survival data. Although limitations on follow-up periods are explained in the text, graphic extrapolation beyond the period of follow-up provides a misleading impression of differences in survival for the two surgical treatment groups. These graphic extrapolations are disconcerting because (1) length of follow-up appears to differ for the two treatment groups, and (2) at least two studies[14, 24] report no relative survival benefit with prophylactic LND after 8 or 9 years of follow-up.

Elimination of the factors that influence patient-physician selection of surgical procedure can only be achieved by conducting randomized prospective trials. The survival results of two randomized prospective trials examining the relationship between prophylactic LND and survival have been recently published and may be considered in further detail.

The Mayo Clinic prospective randomized study, undertaken in 1972, has accrued 171 patients with clinical stage I melanoma.[16, 17] Patients with invasive cutaneous melanoma of the extremities or trunk (except midline lesions) were assigned to one of three treatment groups: WLE alone, WLE with delayed LND (DLND) (2 to 3 months after WLE), and WLE with immediate (LND). Although patients were randomized to these groups, the WLE group was weighted with older patients, patients with deeper lesions, and those with more nodular growth patterns, suggesting that this group had a slight survival disadvantage at the outset. Comparison of the three treatment groups showed no statistically significant differences in survival or disease-free interval.

Using key prognostic variables identified in a multiple regression analysis, a weighted score was developed ranging from 0 (best prognosis) to 7.9 (worst prognosis). Mean prognostic scores for the three groups were 3.31 (WLE), 2.93 (WLE plus DLND), and 2.80 (WLE plus ILND). An additional analysis with patients stratified by prognostic score revealed similar survival for the three surgical treatment groups.[17]

From September 1967 to January 1974, the WHO Melanoma Group trial accrued 553 cases of clinical stage I melanoma to a randomized prospective study evaluating the influence of prophylactic LND on survival.[24] Patients were dichotomously stratified according to presence or absence of prior excisional biopsy and randomized into two surgical treatment groups. The first group was treated with WLE and prophylactic LND; the second group was treated with WLE and only required therapeutic LND if lymph nodes later became clinically suspicious for metastases. To facilitate identification of draining lymph node groups, the study group was restricted to patients with melanomas of the extremity. A small fraction of the study population had primary melanoma with Clark levels of I or II (4.6%) and Breslow depth less than 1.0 mm (9.5%). Nearly 90% of the patient group had lesions of Clark level III, with 61% of tumors measuring between 1.0 and 3.9 mm in Breslow depth. About 7% of this study population had primary melanoma with Clark level V; 31% had tumors at least 4 mm deep. Patients were equally distributed between the two treatment groups by sex, microstage, age, and diameter of the melanoma. The results of this study showed no improvement in 5- or 10-year survival rates for patients randomized to receive prophylactic LND. In addition, the investigators found that survival calculated from the time of prophylactic LND was similar for patients whose LND was performed therapeutically in response to clinical suspicion of lymph node metastases. This finding has been reported by other investigators[21] and refutes the notion that the survival advantage conferred by prophylactic LND results from the early removal of subclinical but pathologically positive lymph nodes, preventing increase in regional tumor burden and reducing risk of metastases to distant sites.[8]

Although the results of published randomized prospective studies indicate no survival benefit due to prophylactic LND, the controversy continues. Results of the WHO trial have been challenged on several grounds, including failure specifically to assess the value of LND in a group at intermediate risk of relapse.[8] Balch[8] has conducted a reanalysis of the WHO data using 40% of the originally identified cases for whom complete clinical and pathologic information was available. Multivariate analysis identified ulceration and tumor thickness as key prognostic factors in this patient subset. On the basis of this analysis, ulceration status and six categories of tumor thickness were combined to create low-, intermediate-, and high-risk patient groups. An analysis of survival rates in the intermediate-risk category revealed improved survival of borderline significance among patients with LND. The authors suggest that the survival benefit in this subgroup was obscured in the overall analysis conducted by the WHO investigators. In fact, the post hoc development of an intermediate risk category comprising a combination of specific levels of risk factors could have introduced, by chance, a spurious association between LND and survival. In this context, the borderline probability level corresponding to the association between LND and survival is not persuasive of a true relationship between LND and survival in this population.

Although the hope of improving patient survival provides the primary rationale for performing prophylactic LND, the usefulness of this procedure in the evaluation and staging of melanoma must also be considered. Data from the WHO study indicate that about half of patients with clinical stage I disease who subsequently develop recurrent disease will relapse first in the regional nodes. In this group, the presence of regional metastases is a predictor of survival outcome. In addition, survival rates differ according to the number of lymph nodes involved with tumor or the presence of tumor limited to microscopic metastases.[11, 27–30] It is also true, however, that about half of patients with clinical stage I disease who relapse will have recurrence simultaneously at regional and distant sites or will develop distant metastases without evidence of lymph node metastases. For these patients, prophylactic LND is not useful as a prognostic variable.

Unfortunately, adjuvant therapies currently available offer little hope of altering patient prognosis.[35, 36] In this context, even for patients who relapse first in the regional lymph nodes, the discovery of lymph node tumor has limited usefulness as a harbinger of distant metastases. However, LND is valuable for determining the presence and extent of regional metastases for randomized trials of potential new adjuvant therapies.

As is true of any surgical procedure, a certain fraction of patients undergoing LND will experience untoward complications. Morbidity associated with regional LND differs for axillary and inguinal sites and with invasiveness of the surgical procedure. Complications arising from axillary LND occur in less than 10% of surgical patients and include hematoma, seroma, cellulitis, permanent edema of the involved extremity, and slough.[12, 37, 38] These complications occur more frequently among patients with inguinal LNDs. In addition, inguinal LND can result in the development of abscess and phlebitis with associated increased risk for pulmonary embolism. In the Mayo Clinic series, lymphedema occurred in 26% and seroma developed in 12% of patients with LND. Although Holmes et al.[12] reported the absence of permanent arm edema in a series of 126 axillary node dissections, disability from leg edema secondary to inguinal node dissection occurred in approximately 20% of surgical patients.[37, 38] Of those suffering from leg edema, major disability causing impairment of work performance and interference with daily routine was noted for eight of 18 patients.[12]

Conclusions

Does Prophylactic LND Improve Survival of Patients With Clinical Stage I Cutaneous Melanoma?

Theoretical support for the use of prophylactic LND among patients with clinical stage I melanoma of intermediate depth arises from two assumptions: (1) melanoma disseminates through the regional lymphatics, and (2) removal of occult metastases present in the draining lymph node groups prevents or slows the spread of disease. The dissemination of melanoma is clearly not mediated solely by the lymphatics. As previously cited, only half of patients in clinical stage I who develop recurrent disease will relapse first in the regional lymph nodes. Whether better tools for the detection of microscopic regional disease might reveal tumor cells in most or all patients who later develop distant metastases is currently an unanswerable question. Several nonrandomized studies support survival benefit with prophylactic LND among patients with clinical stage I melanoma who have tumors of intermediate depth. However, these studies are subject to sources of bias inherent to nonrandomized methodology. Results of the retrospective and nonrandomized prospective studies examining this issue have not been confirmed by randomized prospective investigations designed to evaluate the relationship between LND and survival.

Does Prophylactic LND Improve Control of Regional Disease?

Removal of regional nodes is effective for the control of disease at that site. It is clear, however, that a certain percentage of patients with clinical stage I disease will relapse at distant sites regardless of the status of regional disease. Furthermore, it is not clear that prophylactic LND is more effective for controlling regional disease than is therapeutic LND. Data from at least two studies suggest that survival subsequent to LND is similar for patients with positive node status whether identified at prophylactic or therapeutic LND.[16, 28] Given patient compliance with follow-up examinations allowing frequent evaluation of node status, LND can be performed therapeutically for those patients who may benefit from this procedure without subjecting patients who cannot benefit from LND to the morbidity associated with this surgery. It is our clinical impression that regional disease may ultimately be better controlled by prophylactic surgery, but this requires further study.

Does Prophylactic LND Help Identify High-Risk Individuals Who Might Benefit From Adjuvant Therapy?

For patients in stage I who relapse first at the regional lymph nodes, the number of lymph nodes involved with metastases is a prognostic factor for survival. However, the unavailability of effective adjuvant therapy for patients at risk for distant metastases limits the application of the prognostic information provided by LND to study settings for new potential adjuvant programs.

Does Prophylactic LND Provide Pathologic Material That Can Be Developed Into Therapeutic Agents?

This is an intriguing question for further investigation. The development and implementation of technologies allowing production of lymphokine activated killer cells, tumor infiltrating lymphocytes, human monoclonal antibodies, and antigenic preparations for vaccination remain, at this time, a hope for the future. Although the exploration of these treatment modalities relies on access to tissue specimens, current investigation is limited and does not warrant routine LND for clinical stage I melanoma. Physicians involved in surgical decisions and treatment of patients with melanoma should be aware of the specimen requirements of ongoing research so that dissected tissue can be processed for use in the development of therapeutic modalities. However, the benefits of these modalities must be established before LND is incorporated as standard surgical treatment for these purposes.

What Is the Morbidity Associated With Prophylactic LND?

The morbidity associated with LND includes both local and surgical complications. Local morbidity of node dissection includes seroma, hematoma, cellulitis, abscess, phlebitis, slough, and lymphedema. Surgical morbidity is slightly increased by additional risk for pulmonary embolism when LND reduces capacity for ambulation. Complications arising from LND occur in approximately 10% to 20% of patients. In light of evidence for similar post-surgical survival among patients receiving prophylactic or therapeutic LND, the risks associated with this surgery are unnecessarily incurred when LND is performed without clinical suspicion of nodal metastases.

The utility of prophylactic LND is currently being examined by two international cooperative randomized prospective trials. The trial conducted by the Intergroup Melanoma Committee of the National Cancer Institute

(NCI) randomizes patients with primary melanomas to one of four groups: (1) 2-cm margin for WLE alone; (2) 4-cm margin for WLE alone; (3) 2-cm margin for WLE plus prophylactic regional LND; (4) 4-cm margin for WLE plus prophylactic regional LND. Stratification variables for this study are depth, location of primary tumor, and ulceration. The WHO Melanoma Group trial will evaluate the benefit of prophylactic LND among patients with truncal melanoma and is a sister protocol to the published study evaluating extremity lesions only. In this study, patients will be randomly assigned to WLE or WLE plus prophylactic LND.[8] Whereas the NCI intergroup study focuses on first primary melanoma of 1 to 4 mm, the WHO Melanoma Group is specifically evaluating truncal melanoma exceeding 2 mm in depth.

At present, the evidence for the use of prophylactic LND arises from retrospective and nonrandomized prospective studies, both of which are subject to the influences of various biases. The results of two randomized prospective trials do not confirm the findings of the nonrandomized studies. In addition, the results of several nonrandomized studies refute or provide equivocal evidence for a survival benefit due to prophylactic LND. To conclude, the utility of prophylactic LND remains a controversial issue. The value of prophylactic LND for improving survival among patients with clinical stage I melanoma, or among a subset of these patients, is not yet established. It is hoped that the results of the two ongoing randomized trials will contribute to our knowledge and understanding of the relative merits of prophylactic and therapeutic LND in the treatment of clinical stage I melanoma.

References

1. Block GE, Hartwell SW Jr: Malignant melanoma: A study of 217 cases. *Ann Surg* 1961; 154(suppl):74.
2. Handley WS: The Hunterian lectures on the pathology of melanotic growths in relation to their operative treatment. *Lancet* 1907; 1:927.
3. Stewart DE, Hay LJ, Varco RL: Malignant melanomas: Ninety-two cases treated at the University of Minnesota Hospitals since January 1, 1932.
4. Pack GT, Scharnagel IM, Morfit M: The principle of excision and dissection in continuity for primary and metastatic melanomas of the skin. *Surgery* 1945; 17:849.
5. Luikart S, Kennealey G, Kirkwood J: Randomized phase III trial of vinblastine, bleomycin, and cis-dichlorodiammine-platinum vs. dacarbazine in malignant melanoma. *J Clin Oncol* 1984; 2:164.
6. Kirkwood J, Ernstoff E: The role of interferons in the management of melanoma, in Nathanson L (ed): *Management of Advanced Melanoma.* New York, Churchill Livingstone, Inc, 1986, pp 209–223.
7. Ariel IM: Malignant melanoma of the trunk: A retrospective review of 1128 patients. *Cancer* 1982; 49:1070.

8. Balch CM: Elective lymph node dissection: Pros and cons, in Balch CM, Milton GW (eds): *Cutaneous Melanoma: Clinical Mangement and Treatment Results World Wide.* Philadelphia, JB Lippincott Co, 1985, pp 131–157.
9. Breslow A: Tumor thickness, level of invasion and node dissection in stage I cutaneous melanoma. *Ann Surg* 1975; 182:572.
10. Das Gupta TK: Results of treatment of 269 patients with primary cutaneous melanoma: A 5-year prospective study. *Ann Surg* 1977; 186:201.
11. Fortner JG, Woodruff J, Schottenfeld D: Biostatistical basis of elective node dissection for malignant melanoma. *Ann Surg* 1977; 186:101.
12. Holmes EC, Moseley HS, Morton DL, et al: A rational approach to the surgical management of melanoma. *Ann Surg* 1977; 186:481.
13. Kapelanski DP, Block GE, Kaufman M: Characteristics of the primary lesion of malignant melanoma as a guide to prognosis and therapy. *Ann Surg* 1979; 189:225.
14. Wanebo JH, Woodruff J, Fortner JG: Malignant melanoma of the extremities: A clinicopathologic study using levels of invasion (microstage). *Cancer* 1975; 35:666–676.
15. Balch CM, Soong S-J, Milton GW, et al: A comparison of prognostic factors and surgical results in 1,786 patients wtih localized (stage I) melanoma treated in Alabama, USA and New South Wales, Australia. *Ann Surg* 1982; 196:677.
16. Sim FH, Taylor WF, Pritchard DJ, et al: Lymphadenectomy in the management of stage I malignant melanoma: A prospective randomized study. *Mayo Clin Proc* 1986; 61:697–705.
17. Sim FH, Taylor WF, Ivins JC, et al: A prospective randomized study of the efficacy of routine elective lymphadenectomy in management of malignant melanoma: Preliminary result. *Cancer* 1978; 41:948–956.
18. Blois MS, Sagebiel RW, Tuttle MS, et al: Judging prognosis in malignant melanoma of the skin. *Ann Surg* 1983; 198:200.
19. Roses DF, Harris MN, Hidalgo D, et al: Primary melanoma thickness correlated with regional lymph node metastases. *Arch Surg* 1982; 117:921.
20. Milton GW, Shaw HM, McCarthy WH, et al: Prophylactic lymph node dissection in clinical stage I cutaneous malignant melanoma: Results of surgical treatment in 1319 patients. *Br J Surg* 1982; 69:108–111.
21. Balch CM, Soong S-J, Murad TM, et al: A multifactorial analysis of melanoma: II. Prognostic factors in patients with stage I (localized) melanoma. *Surgery* 1979; 86:343.
22. Bagley FH, Cady B, Lee A, et al: Changes in clinical presentation and management of malignant melanoma. *Cancer* 1981; 47:2126.
23. McCarthy WH, Dobson AJ, Martyn AL, et al: Melanoma in New South Wales, 1970–1976: Surgical therapy and survival. *Aust NZ J Surg* 1982; 52:424–430.
24. Veronesi U, Adamus J, Bandiera DC, et al: Delayed regional lymph node dissection in stage I melanoma of the skin of the lower extremities. *Cancer* 1982; 49:2420–2430.
25. Clark WH Jr, From L, Bernardino EA, et al: The histogenesis and biologic behaviour of primary human malignant melanomas of the skin. *Cancer Res* 1969; 29:705–726.
26. Breslow A: Thickness, cross-sectional areas and depth of invasion in the prognosis of cutaneous melanoma. *Ann Surg* 1970; 172:902–903.

27. Karakousis CP, Seddiq MK, Moore R: Prognostic value of lymph node dissection in malignant melanoma. *Arch Surg* 1980; 115:719.
28. Balch CM, Soong S-J, Murad TM, et al: A multifactorial analysis of melanoma: III. Prognostic factors in melanoma patients with lymph node metastases (stage II). *Ann Surg* 1981; 193:377–388.
29. Callery C, Cochran A, Roe DJ, et al: Factors prognostic for survival in patients with malignant melanoma spread to the regional lymph nodes. *Ann Surg* 1982; 196:69.
30. Cohen MH, Ketcham AS, Felix EL, et al: Prognostic factors in patients undergoing lymphadenectomy for malignant melanoma. *Ann Surg* 1977; 186:635.
31. Cascinelli N, Preda F, Baglini M, et al: Metastatic spread of stage I melanoma of the skin. *Tumori* 1983; 69:449.
32. Klein Baum DG, Kupper LL, Morgenstern H: *Epidemiologic Research*. London, Lifetime Learning Publications, 1982.
33. Schlesselman JJ: *Case-Control Studies*. New York, Oxford University Press, 1982.
34. Kelsey JL, Thompson WD, Evans AS: *Methods in Observational Epidemiology*. New York, Oxford University Press, 1986.
35. Kirkwood JM, Nordlund J, Lerner A, et al: Favorable prognosis of melanoma associated with hypopigmentation (HYP) in a randomized adjuvant trial comparing DTIG-BCG (DB) vs monobenzyl ether of hydroquinone (HQ) vs null (NL) treatment. *Proc Am Soc Clin Oncol* (ASCO 21st Annual Meeting) 1985; 4:149.
36. Ariyan S, Kirkwood JM, Mitchell MS, et al: Intralymphatic and regional surgical adjuvant immunotherapy in high risk melanoma of the extremities. *Surgery* 1982; 92:459–463.
37. Harris MN, Gumport SL, Berman IR, et al: Ilioinguinal lymph node dissection for melanoma. *Surg Gynecol Obstet* 1967; 124:851–865.
38. McCarthy JG, Harajenser CD, Herter FP: The role of groin dissection in the management of melanoma of the lower extremity. *Ann Surg* 1974; 179:156–159.

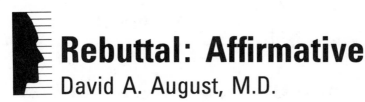

Rebuttal: Affirmative

David A. August, M.D.

Drs. Ernstoff, Titus-Ernstoff, Duray, and Kirkwood conclude their argument against the routine use of ILND in the treatment and evaluation of patients with limited malignant melanoma by stating that "the utility of prophylactic LND remains a controversial issue" and note that completion of the two ongoing randomized trials investigating this issue will contribute to our ability to resolve this controversy. I certainly agree with both of these statements. Our approaches to the controversy differ not so much in conclusion but in emphasis. Nevertheless, it may be helpful to offer a number of comments on their presentation and discussion, and then offer my own answers to the summary questions that they have posed.

Ernstoff et al. emphasize the limitations of retrospective investigations and the sources of bias that may influence the results of such studies. Most would agree that prospective, randomized, single-institution trials represent the gold standard. Nevertheless, this does not a priori invalidate the findings of retrospective or prospective nonrandomized trials, nor should it encourage one to ignore trends identified by such trials. Though not definitive, the studies of Balch, Breslow, and Milton cited by Ernstoff et al. cannot be disregarded. They suggest possible benefit of ILND to significant subsets of patients with melanoma, and these assertions require either confirmation or refutation in subsequent prospective, randomized trials. Conversely, the mere fact that a study is prospective and randomized does not guarantee that the questions addressed will be answered in a definitive and accurate manner. Errors in study design and the nature of patient accrual may prevent acquisition of definitive answers to the questions posed. The WHO and Mayo Clinic prospective, randomized studies were designed to investigate the utility of ILND for patients with clinical stage I melanoma. These studies used only anatomic exclusions among the well-recognized prognostic factors. As such, neither study addresses selective application of ILND. The subgroup analysis used in the WHO study was retrospective as there was no prerandomization stratification of patients according to prognostic features. Thus, the subgroup analysis is inconclusive. In both studies, most patients, by virtue of tumor location, sex, and microstage were among those perhaps least likely to benefit from ILND. Thus, these patient populations were not ideally suited for elucidating a more selective role for ILND.

I quibble with the statistics quoted by Ernstoff et al. regarding the morbidity associated with regional LND. From data collected by Urist and others and similar data quoted in the surgical literature, the incidence of post-LND disability ought to be less than 10%. By further exempting those patients at high risk for developing a postdissection complication (obese and aged patients) from regional lymphadenectomy, these morbidity rates may be reduced even further.

Finally, let me address the summary questions that my colleagues posed.

Does prophylactic LND improve survival of patients with clinical stage I cutaneous melanoma? My colleagues have stated the issues concisely. We agree that the nonrandomized studies supporting survival benefits with ILND are suggestive but subject to sources of bias inherent to nonrandomized methology. That these suggestive results have not been confirmed by the published prospective, randomized investigations is not surprising. These studies were not specifically designed to answer this question for specific subgroups of patients with malignant melanoma.

Does prophylactic LND improve control of regional disease? Ernstoff et al. note that ILND does not help all patients with clinical stage I disease, not even all of those in whom nodal disease is found. They likewise note that ILND may not be more effective than DLND for controlling regional disease. In the case supporting ILND, I have presented data that indicate that ILND is potentially beneficial to most patients with malignant melanoma. The challenge remains to identify criteria that will permit prospective selection of the patients who will benefit from ILND and thus should undergo the procedure.

Does prophylactic LND help identify high-risk individuals who might benefit from adjuvant therapy? We are in agreement that though the presence of regional lymph node metastases and the number of nodes involved are prognostic for survival, given the unavailability of effective adjuvant therapies this information is not currently clinically relevant. It is of importance, however, within study settings investigating new adjuvant programs.

Does prophylactic LND provide pathologic material that can be developed into therapeutic agents? Such a possibility offers a strong indication for the use of ILND within appropriate study settings. The benefits of these modalities must be established, however, before ILND should be routinely undertaken for this purpose.

What is the morbidity associated with prophylactic LND? Determination of an acceptable complication rate for ILND cannot be made until the extent of benefit conferred by ILND is more accurately established. Regional lymphadenectomy may be carried out with morbidity rates under 10%, and this is acceptable for a potentially lifesaving procedure.

I can only agree with Drs. Ernstoff, Titus-Ernstoff, Duray, and Kirkwood that it is the results of ongoing randomized trials that will ultimately define the appropriate role for ILND in the treatment of patients with malignant melanoma.

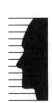

Rebuttal: Negative

Marc S. Ernstoff, M.D., Linda Titus-Ernstoff, Paul H. Duray, M.D., and John M. Kirkwood, M.D.

We believe that there is general agreement for ILND among patients with melanoma with clinical stage II disease. For patients with stage III disease, LND may occasionally be useful for symptomatic relief. In addition, prophylactic LND is useful for the disease staging of patients who may be eligible for experimental treatment. The continuing area of controversy concerns the therapeutic usefulness of prophylactic LND among patients with clinical stage I disease.

We agree that very real differences exist in survival rates for patients with localized disease vs. patients with regional disease. It is a leap of faith, however, to infer that these survival differences support the effectiveness of prophylactic LND for the treatment of clinical stage I disease. Although the importance of preventing regional and distant metastases provides strong incentive for aggressive intervention, randomized trials do not support the usefulness of prophylactic LND for preventing metastatic disease.

The belief that LND can cure patients with clinical stage I disease is based on the assumption that melanoma disseminates in an orderly, sequential fashion, passing first through the regional lymph nodes and then to distant sites.[1] There is strong evidence to suggest that this is not always the case. Of those patients with clinical stage I disease destined to develop metastatic disease, melanoma will recur first at distant sites for about 30% and will recur simultaneously at regional and distant sites in about 20%.[2] The potential value of LND is limited to the fraction of patients whose disease will recur first in the regional lymph nodes, representing about 50% of patients destined for disease recurrence and 20% of the total group with clinical stage I disease. The question remains whether prophylactic LND is of therapeutic value for this 20% in clinical stage I. Equivalent survival periods reported for patients with positive nodes identified either at the time of prophylactic LND or at the time of DLND[2, 3] provide strong evidence that ILND does not confer survival advantage. Randomized studies designed to evaluate the usefulness of prophylactic LND have failed to detect survival benefit for patients receiving this treatment.

The results of nonrandomized studies aimed at evaluating the usefulness of prophylactic LND are varied and equivocal. One must suspect that selection biases operating in these studies tend to create spurious results favoring prophylactic LND. Depending on surgical acumen, patients with good prognoses may be more likely than patients with poor prognoses to receive prophylactic surgery. The existence of this influence is suggested by the somewhat more favorable assessments of prophylactic LND arising in the setting of nonrandomized studies susceptible to the effects of selection bias. It is interesting that several authors maintain support for prophylactic LND in the presence of limited statistical evidence in their own studies. The discrepancy between the statistical results of these studies and the conclusions drawn by some of the investigators underscores the widespread entrenchment of belief in the utility of prophylactic LND.

Randomized clinical trials offer the optimal approach to examining survival outcomes associated with different methods of treatment. The purpose of randomization is to distribute equally among treatment categories patients from all prognostic subsets of a larger but defined diagnostic group. It is unnecessary, and often cumbersome, to stratify patients by prognostic factors before randomization.[4, 5] The effectiveness of randomization for producing a balanced distribution of patients can be evaluated post hoc by examining the distribution of prognostic variables in the treatment groups.[4] The post hoc evaluation of the distribution of prognostic factors in the WHO trial revealed that randomization without stratification had successfully produced a balance of prognostic factors in the two surgical treatment groups.

The randomized clinical trials conducted by WHO and the Mayo Clinic failed to demonstrate overall survival differences in the surgical treatment groups. In addition, single-factor stratified analyses were conducted to examine survival outcomes within prognostic categories. In the Mayo trial, risk "scores" were created post hoc using prognostic variables identified in regression analyses. In both studies, analyses conducted by single prognostic factors failed to reveal differences in survival for the surgical treatment groups. A reevaluation of the WHO data conducted by Balch et al.[1] demonstrated no survival advantage associated with prophylactic LND in any single prognostic category, including ulceration, that had not been evaluated in the original analysis. Balch et al.[1] also reanalyzed the WHO data and found that immediate LND offered a survival advantage to a particular "intermediate-risk" subgroup identified by examining combined categories of ulceration and five levels of tumor depth. The post hoc development of multiple subgroups for statistical analysis increases the probability of observing spurious findings arising from random sampling variation.[4, 6] For this reason, the results of multiple comparisons must be subjected to stringent probability levels for the evaluation of statistical significance.[4, 6] Because Balch et al. evaluated several combinations of prognostic factors to create an intermediate risk group, the "marginal" significance level associated with this subgroup is not statistically meaningful.

In the WHO trial, participants were restricted to patients with tumors of the extremity. Although these patients generally have better survival than patients with tumors of the head or trunk, this advantage was necessarily distributed equally between the two surgical treatment groups. More to the point, this restriction facilitated the identification of draining lymph node groups for surgical removal and consequently allowed the evaluation of prophylactic LND among those patients who were most likely to benefit from this procedure.

Despite specific analyses directed at examining survival outcome with stratification on prognostic factors, survival differences for surgical treatment methods were not detected by either randomized trial. Although it is possible that the failure to identify differences in treatment outcomes of the controversial intermediate-risk subgroup is due to inadequate sample sizes in these studies, it is unlikely that substantial differences in treatment outcomes would escape detection.

It is conceivable that prophylactic LND benefits a small fraction of patients with clinical stage I melanoma. In the future, large, randomized trials directed at the evaluation of this treatment among patients in the intermediate-risk category may succeed in demonstrating survival advantage for the recipients of prophylactic LND. The development of technology allowing the identification of patients most likely to benefit from prophylactic LND would be helpful in creating prognostic categories for future trials and potentially for therapeutic decisions. Currently, diagnostic technology and statistical support for the therapeutic utility of prophylactic LND are not available. The randomized trials best suited to the examination of this issue do not provide evidence of survival advantage associated with prophylactic LND. In the absence of compelling evidence demonstrating an extended survival advantage among patients receiving prophylactic LND, it seems unreasonable to subject large numbers of patients to this potentially morbid and unnecessary surgery.

References

1. Balch CM, Cascinelli N, Milton GW, et al: Elective lymph node dissection: Pros and cons, in Balch CM, Milton GW (eds): *Cutaneous Melanoma: Clinical Management and Treatment Results World Wide*. Philadelphia, JB Lippincott Co, 1985, pp 131–157.
2. Veronesi U, Adamus J, Bandiera DC, et al: Delayed regional lymph node dissection in stage I melanoma of the skin of the lower extremities. *Cancer* 1982; 49:2420–2430.
3. Balch CM, Soong S-J, Murad TM, et al: A multifactorial analysis of melanoma: II. Prognostic factors in patients with stage I (localized) melanoma. *Surgery* 1979; 86:343.
4. Colton T: *Statistics in Medicine*. Boston, Little, Brown & Co, 1974.
5. Meinert CL: *Clinical Trials: Design, Conduct and Analysis*. New York, Oxford University Press, 1986.
6. Keppel G: *Design and Analysis: A Researcher's Handbook*. Englewood Cliffs, NJ, Prentice-Hall International Inc, 1973.

Editor's Comments
Thomas P. Duffy, M.D.

Both parties to the controversy regarding immediate lymph node dissection (ILND) for clinical stage I cutaneous melanoma agree that there is a population of such patients, admittedly small, who may benefit from ILND. However, randomized, prospective studies have failed to demonstrate any survival advantage for the procedure when employed indiscriminately for management of clinical stage I disease. This therapeutic failure must imply that the identification of patients potentially curable with ILND eludes detection and highlights the need to develop methods to demonstrate metastases before they are clinically evident. Capitalizing upon membrane markers unique to melanoma cells may provide a means of detection as well as a means of delivering chemotherapy to metastatic areas.

The quandary regarding the proper use of surgery in cutaneous melanoma echoes the debates which raged in the management of breast malignancy.

A more restrained attitude regarding surgical intervention is now in place following the recognition that breast cancer is frequently a systemic disease on presentation. Radical mastectomy has been usurped by lumpectomy with adjuvant treatments of chemotherapy or irradiation. Better understanding of the basic pathophysiology of a disease has dictated a less invasive management of the lesion.

In a parallel fashion, less may constitute more in the management of cutaneous melanoma. But the fact that a minority of patients with potentially curable disease will be deprived of that cure is unsettling and disturbing. All would agree that studies are necessary to permit the identification of this population in the future. It is also hoped that these same studies will provide the means to make the current debate outdated because a more physiologic approach to the disease has been identified.

Restriction of Dietary Protein Is the Critical Component in Altering the Progression of Renal Failure in Patients With Chronic Renal Disease

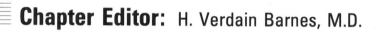

Chapter Editor: H. Verdain Barnes, M.D.

Affirmative: Thomas Hostetter, M.D.
Associate Professor of Medicine, Director,
Section of Renal Disease, Department of
Medicine, University of Minnesota Hospitals,
Minneapolis, Minnesota

Anthony C. Wooley, M.D.
Instructor, Renal Division, Department of
Medicine, University of Minnesota Hospitals,
Minneapolis, Minnesota

Negative: Allen C. Alfrey, M.D.
Professor of Medicine, Department of
Medicine, University of Colorado, Health
Sciences Center; Chief, Renal Medicine,
Veterans Administration Medical Center,
Denver, Colorado

Debates in Medicine 1:222–247, 1988
© 1988, Year Book Medical Publishers, Inc.
0887-218X/88/01-222-247-$04.00

Affirmative

Thomas H. Hostetter, M.D., and
Anthony C. Wooley, M.D.

Established chronic renal insufficiency tends to progress to end-stage renal failure regardless of the initial cause of renal damage. Even after the apparent initial cause of renal injury is removed, for example, after acute cortical necrosis or the correction of obstructive uropathy, renal function often continues to decline. This progressive nature of renal disease has led to a search for some final common pathway of renal injury. Experimental and clinical evidence points to a prominent role for intrarenal hemodynamic changes mediated by dietary protein as such a pathway.

Central to understanding the response to chronic renal injury is the intact nephron hypothesis; the idea that diseased kidneys and the individual nephron units in diseased kidneys can continue to function in a physiologically predictable manner. Virtually all chronic renal diseases result in striking structural and functional heterogeneity within the kidney. Single-nephron glomerular filtration rates (GFRs) may vary from less than to several times greater than those seen in normal kidneys. Tubular function, and in particular the reabsorption of water and electrolytes, remains tightly coupled to single-nephron GFRs such that nephrons with high GFRs will have proportionally elevated rates of fluid and solute reabsorption. Thus, *glomerulotubular balance* is maintained in the diseased kidney across a greatly expanded range of single-nephron GFRs.

In keeping with retained physiologic function of surviving nephron units, striking compensatory hypertrophy and hyperfunction occur. This has been recognized for over 100 years as pathologists have noted hypertrophy of undiseased nephrons in a variety of kidney diseases. Following removal of one kidney in animals or humans, striking growth of the remaining kidney occurs. New nephron units are not formed; rather, there is hypertrophy and to a lesser extent hyperplasia of existing nephrons, in particular of the metabolically active proximal tubular cells. As evidence of early anabolic processes, a substantial increase in the RNA content of the remaining kidney can be seen within 12 hours following uninephrectomy. Compensatory renal growth is accompanied by striking hyperfunction at both single-nephron and whole-kidney levels. In humans, the GFR in the remaining kidney rises within 24 hours after uninephrectomy and reaches 60% to 90% of the preoperative two-kidney value by 4 months. Striking increases in renal blood flow occur within days of uninephrectomy, suggesting that hemodynamic events occur early in the process of hyperfunction and hypertrophy.

In experimental animals, hyperfunction can be studied at a single-nephron level in various models of renal disease. One such model that has been studied extensively is so-called remnant kidney disease. In this model, rats undergo removal of one kidney and infarction or surgical removal of a variable portion of the remaining kidney, leaving from 5% to 50% of the original renal mass. Such animals undergo marked growth and hyperfunction in the remaining remnant kidney, initially tending to preserve renal function. However, such compensatory hyperfunction may in the long run be detrimental in that these rats develop a progressive renal disease characterized by systemic hypertension, proteinuria, and, eventually, progressive azotemia. Pathologically remnant kidneys initially undergo glomerular enlargement followed by focal and segmental glomerulosclerosis and a prominent interstitial inflammatory infiltrate, changes seen in most severe chronic renal diseases in humans.

Single-nephron GFR and its determinants may be measured or derived by micropuncture techniques in experimental animals. Glomerular ultrafiltration may be expressed as the Starling relationship, single-nephron GFR = $K_f (\Delta P - \Delta \pi)$, where K_f, the ultrafiltration coefficient, represents the permeability properties of the glomerulus, its filtration surface, and its surface area, and ΔP and $\Delta \pi$ represent Starling's forces across the glomerular capillary wall: the hydraulic pressure gradient and the oncotic pressure gradient, respectively. Because the concentration of protein is greater within the capillary lumen, the resultant oncotic gradient tends to retard ultrafiltration. Although not explicit in this equation, the glomerular plasma flow rate, designated Q_A, is also an important determinant of glomerular filtration, because higher capillary plasma flows tend to reduce the mean glomerular capillary oncotic pressure gradient and thereby increase single-nephron GFR. Micropuncture studies of rats with a variety of experimental renal disease, including the remnant kidney, glomerulonephritis, hypertension, and diabetic nephropathy, have all shown some common glomerular hemodynamic features. Glomerular capillary flow is often increased, even by two to three times that of normal nephrons. Even more consistently, glomerular capillary pressure and the transcapillary hydraulic pressure gradient are also increased. In the remnant kidney model, the amount of renal tissue removed or destroyed is directly proportional to the degree of elevation of glomerular capillary blood flow and single-nephron GFR. The major renal resistance vessels and, hence, the major intrarenal determinants of blood flow are the afferent and efferent arterioles of the glomerulus. It is primarily vasodilatation of the afferent arteriole in the hyperfiltering nephron that leads to glomerular hyperperfusion (increased Q_A), hypertension (increased PGC), and hyperfiltration (increased single-nephron GFR).

The specific signals that cause the glomerulus to vasodilate, hyperperfuse, and hyperfilter are not completely understood, but dietary protein clearly plays an integral role. Chronic protein feeding in experimental animals leads to increased renal growth. In humans, hyperalimentation with large quantities of amino acids has caused striking increases in kidney size. In normal humans or animals, a protein meal can cause as much as a 40% increase in renal blood flow and GFR. Such changes are sustained in long-term protein feeding. These changes are due to protein itself and not an accompanying nutrient, in that similar increases in renal blood flow and GFR are seen with amino acid infusions or by the oral or intravenous administration of glycine. Metabolic byproducts of protein appear unimportant, as renal blood flow and GFR are increased within 5 minutes of starting an amino acid infusion. Further, dogs fed urea, sulfate, or acid in amounts equivalent to those produced by the catabolism of a protein meal do not exhibit these effects.

The mechanism by which proteins or amino acids cause renal hyperemia and hyperfiltration has not been elucidated. Amino acids infused directly into the isolated perfused kidney have only a small effect on GFR, suggesting that some humoral factors stimulated by amino acids may be involved. Glucagon or some other gastrointestinal hormone has been implicated by some studies. Glucagon is released after protein ingestion and can increase renal blood flow or GFR. Furthermore, somatostatin, which inhibits the secretion of glucagon and several other peptide hormones, can completely block the renal response to protein ingestion or amino acid infusion. However, experiments trying to establish glucagon as the mediator of this process have met with mixed results. In one interesting experiment the direct infusion of glucagon into the renal artery of dogs had no effect on renal blood flow or GFR; however, infusion of glucagon into the portal vein resulted in 25% increase in renal blood flow and GFR. These results suggest that glucagon causes the elaboration of a hepatic hormone, which in turn induces renal vasodilation, hyperemia, and hyperfiltration.

Prostaglandins may be the specific mediators of glomerular vasodilation. Whole-kidney and glomerular production of the vasodilator prostaglandin E_2 is increased in several models of chronic renal disease, and the prostaglandin inhibitor indomethacin reduces glomerular plasma flow and single-nephron GFR in the remnant model. Further, prostaglandin E excretion is increased by raising the intake of dietary protein.

Dietary protein also stimulates renin secretion; hence, a role for angiotensin II in mediating hyperfiltration in remnant glomeruli has been proposed. Angiotensin II has a relatively specific effect in the glomerulus, causing primarily efferent arteriolar constriction. Such postglomerular vasoconstriction increases single-nephron GFR by increasing intracapillary pressure. In both remnant kidney disease and experimental diabetes, angiotensin inhibition with converting enzyme inhibitors normalizes glomerular capillary pressure and markedly attenuates renal injury. Preliminary studies of converting enzyme inhibitors in human renal disease suggest a beneficial role, although long-term trials have not been done. Recent evidence has demonstrated that protein restriction in humans with renal disease decreases plasma renin activity. Hence, part of the effect of dietary protein on renal hemodynamics may be by stimulating the intrarenal renin-angiotensin axis, resulting in relative postglomerular constriction and glomerular capillary hypertension.

The mechanisms that cause acute renal hemodynamic changes after protein ingestion appear also to be responsible for the sustained hyperperfusion and hyperfiltration seen in animals with chronic renal diseases. Manipulation of dietary protein in the remnant model of kidney failure produces striking changes in glomerular hemodynamics. Figure 1 shows the effects of reduction of dietary protein content from 24% to 6% on single-nephron GFR, glomerular capillary plasma flow, and mean glomerular capillary pressure in rats subjected to 90% nephrectomy. Marked increases in glomerular plasma flow, capillary pressure, and GFR are seen in the remnant animals fed 24% protein. These values are maintained at normal or near-normal levels in remnant rats fed 6% protein. Similar blunting of glomerular hypertension and hyperperfusion has been shown in remnant glomeruli several months after renal ablation, even when protein restriction is instituted well after remnant kidney disease is established. The restoration of normal glomerular hemodynamics by protein restriction in remnant kidney disease is associated with decreased proteinuria, preservation of renal function, attenuation of histologic renal injury, and improved survival. After 1⅓ nephrectomy, a relatively low-grade degree of renal abla-

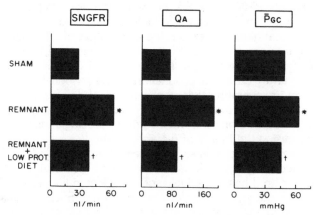

FIG 1.
Average increases in SNGFR, Q_A, and $\bar{P}_{GC}$ in remnant glomeruli of rats undergoing 90% nephrectomy 7 days previously *(middle row)* relative to values in sham-operated control rats *(top row)*, and 90% nephrectomy rats fed low (6%) protein chow *(bottom row)*. Animals in *top* and *middle rows* were fed 24% protein diets. (From Brenner BM: Nephron adaptation to renal injury or ablation. *Am J Physiol* 1985; 249:F324-F337. Reproduced by permission.)

tion, at 8 months rats fed a 40% protein diet excreted 57 mg of protein in the urine per 24 hours and histologically had global sclerosis of 37.2% of glomeruli. In contrast, rats fed a 6% protein diet excreted only 16 mg of protein per 24 hours and had only 17% global sclerosis. In this study the diets had identical amounts of vitamins, trace elements, and minerals added and were similar in phosphate content.

Indeed, dietary protein restriction has been shown to reduce renal injury and retard the progression of renal insufficiency in virtually every experimental model of renal disease, including models of diabetic nephropathy, lupus nephritis, mineralocorticoid hypertension, and chronic glomerulonephritis. Recent studies have shown a beneficial effect on experimental tubulointerstitial disease as well. Besides studies of dietary protein manipulation, a variety of other evidence implicates glomerular hypertension in chronic nephron injury. In spontaneously hypertensive rats, in rats with mineralocorticoid-induced hypertension, and in experimental diabetes, glomerulosclerosis occurs only when glomerular capillary hypertension is present. As previously stated, angiotensin converting enzyme inhibitors can normalize glomerular capillary pressure by relaxation of the efferent arteriole in both remnant kidney disease and experimental diabetes and, in so doing, greatly attenuate renal injury. In numerous other studies, when glomerular capillary pressure has been manipulated, renal injury has responded in the expected fashion. Hence, the bulk of evidence suggests that glomerular capillary hypertension is of major importance in the progression of chronic renal disease and that dietary protein intake can control the level of capillary pressure.

The mechanism by which increased glomerular capillary pressure causes renal injury is unknown. In analogy to current theories of the pathogenesis of atherosclerosis, glomerular capillary hypertension may lead to injury to endothelial or other component cells of the glomerulus with secondary activation of platelets, clotting mechanisms, and inflammatory or mitogenic mediators. Indeed, there is evidence that anticlotting or antiplatelet drugs are beneficial in experimental, and in some cases human, renal disease. With reference to the atherosclerosis analogy, lowering cholesterol levels with the pharmacologic agents lovastatin (Mevinolin) or clofibrate reduces renal injury in the remnant kidney independent of hemodynamic factors, suggesting that hyperlipidemia may play a role in the pathogenesis of experimental renal disease. Another proposed mechanism by which glomerular hypertension could lead to renal damage is from increased transcapillary protein flux, leading to mesangial proliferation and/or direct mesangial injury.

Nonhemodynamic effects of protein may also be important in propagating progression. For example, oxygen free radicals could potentially mediate cellular damage in chronic renal failure (CRF). Because glomerulotubular balance is retained, hyperfiltration obligates increased sodium reabsorption per nephron. As this is the major energy-requiring process of the nephron, increased oxygen consumption would be expected. Aerobic metabolism produces oxygen free radicals that, if present in sufficient concentration, can damage lipid membranes, proteins, and nucleic acids and lead to cell death. Hence, dietary protein restriction could, by decreasing renal oxygen demand, limit such cellular injury.

Adaptive increases in other tubular functions, in particular ammonia production, also occur. The resultant increase in intrarenal ammonia can activate the alternative complement pathway by the nonenzymatic amidization of C3. Amidized C3 can serve as a convertase, activating the membrane attack complex and stimulating inflammatory mediators. Because protein restriction lowers dietary acid production and ammonia production, this may represent yet another beneficial nonhemodynamic effect of protein restriction. Figure 2 depicts schematically a hypothetical model of the interactions of various forces thought to be important in this phenomenon.

The degree of reduction of renal mass necessary to cause injury to remaining nephrons is unknown. Focal glomerulosclerosis has been reported to occur with increased frequency in patients who have unilateral renal agenesis or who have had a unilateral nephrectomy in the distant past. There is an increased prevalence of sclerotic glomeruli in rats after uninephrectomy. Increasing attention in recent years has been paid to renal transplant donors, who are usually carefully evaluated for the presence of any renal disease or hypertension and, hence, represent a group of normal individuals who undergo unilateral nephrectomy. For the most part longitudinal studies have demonstrated a benign course for these donors; however, some studies have reported an increased incidence of hypertension and elevated levels of urinary protein excretion. Furthermore, follow-up rarely exceeds 20 years' duration, which is not sufficient to answer firmly the question of whether any of these individuals will eventually develop clinically significant renal disease. Focal sclerosis may also occur with increased frequency in morbidly obese patients, a situation where there may be an increased demand per nephron based not on a reduction in nephron number but rather on an increase in body mass and presumably in dietary intake of protein as well. Rather than a threshold for this phenomenon, a continuum may exist such that the greater the reduction in renal mass at a given level of protein intake, the more severe the hemodynamic glomerular changes and the more rapid the development of renal injury. This view has been used to explain the gradual decline in GFR and increase in the number of sclerotic glomeruli seen with normal aging in western civilization.

There is substantial evidence for a pivotal role of dietary protein in the progression of human renal disease as well. Several studies demonstrate a beneficial effect of protein restriction in human renal diseases. Normally about 0.6 gm of protein per kilogram of body weight per day is required

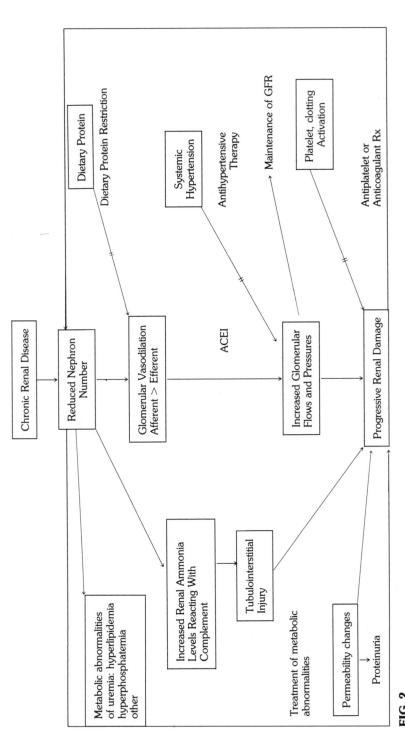

FIG 2.
Schematized, hypothetical view of factors related to progression of renal disease. Note the self-perpetuating nature of the process, whereby reduced nephron number, causing glomerular hypertension, leads to progressive injury and further nephron loss. Potential points of intervention include dietary protein restriction, angiotensin converting enzyme inhibition (ACE I), antiplatelet or anticlotting drugs, antihypertensive therapy, and treatment of metabolic abnormalities such as hyperphosphatemia and hyperlipidemia.

TABLE 1.
Selected Clinical Studies of Protein Restriction in Renal Failure*

	Rosman et al, *Lancet* 1984; 2:1291	Mitch et al, *N Engl J Med* 1984; 311:623	Mascio et al, *Kidney Int* 1983; 24:5273	Williams et al, *Proceedings of the Ninth International Congress on Nephrology,* 1984, p 318A
No. of patients	228 (149 followed up > 18 mo)	24	53 + 40 controls	47
Type of study	Prospective, randomized, controlled	Prospective, uncontrolled	Prospective, historical controls only	Prospective, uncontrolled
Renal function at start of study	Creatinine clearance, 10–60 ml/min	Serum creatinine, 5.2–16.8 mg/dl	Serum creatinine, 1.55–6.7 mg/dl	Mean serum creatinine, 10 mg/dl
Diet	With creatinine clearance of 10–30 ml/min, 0.4 gm/kg/day protein; creatinine clearance of 31–60 ml/min, 0.6 gm/kg/day	20–30 gm/day protein, EAA + KAA supplements, phosphorus restricted	0.6 gm/kg/day protein, 75% HBV, 750 mg/day phosphorus, 1–1.5 gm/day calcium	0.6 gm/kg/day protein, 320 mg/day phosphorus

Results	Decreased slope of 1/creatinine as a function of time regardless of initial renal function; decreased proteinuria, phosphate excretion; improved survival in protein-restricted group	Of 17 patients with clearly definable prior rates of progression, 10 had decreased slope of 1/creatinine; stable in all others	Decreased slope of 1/creatinine; decreased serum phosphorus	Decreased slope of 1/creatinine in 41 patients
Follow-up, mo	>18	Mean, 20	Mean, 41–44 (latest review of these patients)	Mean, 17
Comments	The largest and the only randomized, controlled study published in this area	Good assessment of nutritional status, which was maintained throughout the study	Ongoing study in Europe; "controls" subsequently added to low-protein-diet group	Of note because of advanced renal disease in many patients

*EAA indicates essential amino acids; KAA, ketoacid analogues of amino acids; HBV, high-biologic-value protein.

to maintain nitrogen balance. Some early studies of dietary protein restriction, while demonstrating slower progression of renal disease, also resulted in negative nitrogen balance. The use of high-biologic-value protein (high proportion of essential amino acids) together with a high calorie content can, in some patients, allow nitrogen balance with a protein intake of 20 to 25 gm/day. Other studies using protein levels of about 0.6 gm/kg/day have also showed significant slowing of the progression of renal disease, usually measured as the reciprocal of the serum creatinine level (proportional to creatinine clearance) as a function of time. Such studies have shown benefit both in patients with mild renal insufficiency (serum creatinine levels, 1.5 to 3.0 mg/dl) and in patients with advanced renal insufficiency with creatinine levels of 10 mg/dl or higher. Maintaining nitrogen balance with low protein intakes supplemented with essential amino acids or ketoacid analogues of amino acids also has shown significant effects on the progression of renal failure. Recently, restriction of dietary protein to 0.6 gm/kg/day in a group of patients with chronic renal transplant rejection resulted in a significant retardation of loss of renal function even though there was no change in immunosuppressant therapy. Although there are methodologic flaws in many of the studies of dietary protein restriction, taken as a whole the literature suggests that a clinically important effect is present. Selected clinical studies are summarized in Table 1.

A criticism of many of these studies has been the lack of control for the level of phosphorus intake; even when phosphorus was not expressly restricted, intake likely fell as protein was restricted. There have been several attempts to try to separate these two variables that suggest that the effects of protein restriction are independent of serum phosphorus or phosphorus intake. In one study, half of the patients eating a low-protein diet were given frequent doses of the phosphate binder aluminum hydroxide. Though the serum phosphorus level in the aluminum hydroxide–supplemented group was below that of controls, there was no difference in the rate of progression. In another study of a low-protein, essential amino acid–supplemented diet, progression was slowed in some patients whose serum phosphorus level increased. In a study of a low-protein plus ketoacid analogue–supplemented diet, the slowing of progression of renal insufficiency was not dependent on the maintenance of a normal serum phosphorus level. In one short-term study of patients with nephrotic-range proteinuria and moderate renal insufficiency, a decrease in proteinuria and improvement in glomerular permselective properties was observed in a low-protein as opposed to a high-protein diet even though the low-protein diet was supplemented to contain the same phosphorus content as the high-protein diet. Several experimental studies have also rigorously divorced the effect of alteration in phosphate intake and/or its levels in plasma and urine from the effect of dietary protein, indicating that protein restriction has an independent and powerful effect on progressive disease. Thus, though severe restriction of dietary phosphorus may limit progressive chronic renal injury, this effect appears to be separate and independent from that of dietary protein restriction.

Bibliography

1. Brenner BM: Nephron adaptation to renal injury or ablation. *Am J Physiol* 1985; 249:F324–F337.
2. Brenner BM, Meyer TW, Hostetter TH: Dietary protein in the progressive nature of kidney disease: The role of hemodynamically mediated glomerular injury and the pathogenesis of progressive glomerular sclerosis in ageing renal ablation and intrinsic renal disease. *N Engl J Med* 1982; 307:652–659.
3. El Nahas AM, Kohls GA: Dietary treatment of chronic renal failure: Ten unanswered questions. *Lancet* 1986; 1:597–600.
4. Hostetter TH: The hyperfiltering glomerulus. *Med Clin North Am* 1984; 68:387–398.
5. Hostetter TH, Meyer TW, Rennke HG, et al: Chronic effects of dietary protein in the rat with intact and reduced renal mass. *Kidney Int* 1986; 30:509–517.
6. Hostetter TH, Olson JL, Rennke HG, et al: Hyperfiltration in remnant nephrons: A potentially adverse response to renal ablation. *Am J Physiol* 1981; 241:F85–F93.
7. Mitch WE: The influence of the diet on the progression of renal insufficiency. *Annu Rev Med* 1984; 35:249–264.

Negative

Allen C. Alfrey, M.D.

Almost half a century ago, dietary protein restriction was shown to exert a protective effect on preserving renal function in experimental renal disease. However, this observation was not greatly extended until the past decade, when interest in dietary manipulation in the treatment of CRF was renewed. This was largely predicated on the fact that it was becoming evident that a large number of patients were receiving renal transplants or long-term dialysis therapy for end-stage renal disease. Not only were these therapeutic modalities far from ideal in that they were associated with considerable mortality and morbidity, but they also resulted in an enormous financial burden on society. The obvious solution to this problem would be to develop a means of either slowing or preventing the progression of CRF to end-stage renal disease. Additional interest in dietary therapy was further renewed when Drs. Hostetter and Brenner suggested a mechanism by which protein restriction could exert its protective effect in one type of experimental renal disease, the remnant kidney model. However, it has subsequently been shown that a variety of different dietary maneuvers including calorie restriction, manipulation of lipid type and content in the diet, and phosphate restriction can have as much protective effect as protein restriction in the preservation of renal function in experimental renal disease. Because of the diverse nature of these various dietary maneuvers, it seems unlikely that they all exert their protective effect through a common mechanism. Of the various dietary manipulations besides protein restriction, phosphate restriction has been the most extensively studied. Also, there has been more controversy regarding what, if any, beneficial effect phosphate restriction has on the preservation of renal function in chronic renal disease.

Dietary phosphate restriction was initially shown to prevent renal functional deterioration, proteinuria, and histologic alterations in the rat remnant kidney model of renal failure in 1978. These studies were subsequently extended in the same model of renal failure to show that even after the disease was well established, dietary phosphate restriction could be effective. Thirty days after the remnant kidney was established, rats were placed on either a normal or phosphate-restricted diet. As can be appreciated in Figure 3, rats maintained on a low-phosphorus diet actually had an improvement in renal function as documented by the fall in plasma creatinine level. In contrast, the rats maintained on the regular diet had progression of their renal failure. There was also a marked reduction in urinary protein excretion in the phosphate-restricted rats.

To extend these observations further, additional studies were performed in another experimental model of CRF, nephrotoxic serum nephritis,

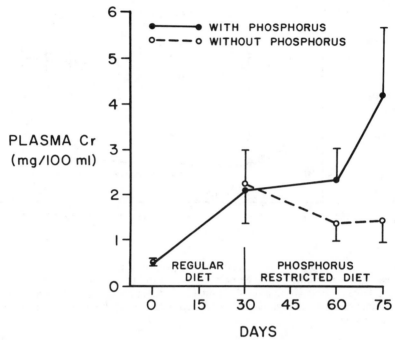

FIG 3.
Plasma creatinine *(Cr)* levels before nephrectomy, 30 days following the establish-
ment of the remnant kidney when the rats were placed on a phosphate-restricted
diet, and at 60 and 75 days during the phosphate-restricted period. (From Alfrey
AC, Karlinsky M, Haut L: Protective effect of phosphate restriction on renal function. *Adv Exp Med Biol* 1980; 128:209. Used by permission.)

which more closely resembles human renal disease. Animals in these experiments were placed on a phosphate-restricted diet 30 days following
the administration of nephrotoxic serum at a time when the autologous
phase of this disease was well established. As found with the remnant kidney model, dietary phosphate restriction prevented functional deterioration
and markedly reduced renal histologic change. However, it did not interfere with immunoglobulin and complement deposition in the glomerulus.
In contrast, the animals with nephrotoxic serum nephritis maintained on a
normal phosphorus diet had a progressive rise in plasma creatinine and
extensive renal histologic alterations. Ultimately, the animals died of uremia (Fig 4).

The major criticisms of these studies have been presented by Laouari
and Kleinknecht, expressing the concern that in the above studies animals
were not pair-fed and therefore other constituents of the diet could also
have varied. To study this possibility, Laouari and Kleinknecht placed rats

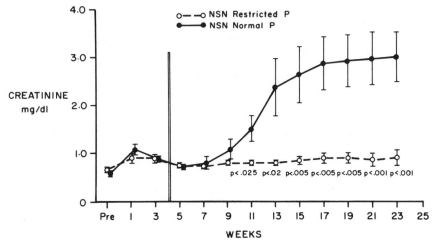

FIG 4.
The effect of phosphate *(P)* restriction on the progression of renal disease in neph-rotoxic serum nephritis *(NSN)* as determined by the measurement of plasma cre-atinine levels. (From Karlinsky M, Haut L, Buddington B, et al: Preservation of renal function in experimental glomerulo nephritis. *Kidney Int* 1980; 17:293. Used by permission.)

with a remnant kidney on 0.2% or 0.5% phosphate diets and pair-fed them with a group of rats on a severely phosphate-restricted diet (0.05%). At the time the study was terminated, 19% of the rats on the 0.05% phos-phate diet had died, whereas 29% and 44% of the pair-fed animals on 0.2% and 0.5% phosphate diets had died. The study was terminated at a time when the mortality was accelerating in the latter two groups of rats, suggesting that if the study had been extended the difference in survival rates would have been even greater between the severely phosphate-re-stricted group and the other two groups of rats. Another deficiency of these studies is the fact that when food consumption was reduced, phosphate intake was also further restricted in the pair-fed rats. This represented an-other uncontrolled variable in these studies. It is of further interest that the histologic alterations were different in the phosphate-restricted rats as com-pared with the nonrestricted animals. In the non–phosphate-restricted groups, tubular lesions and renal parenchymal calcification were much more prominent than in the restricted rats. Because of the various deficien-cies and findings in the above studies, they cannot be considered definitive answers as to whether phosphate restriction alone is protective of renal functional deterioration.

A much better controlled study was carried out by Lumlertgul et al. In this study animals were fed an identical diet and meticulously pair-fed. The adequacy of pair-feeding was documented by showing that urine nitrogen excretion and body weight were not different between the phosphate-restricted animals and nonrestricted animals throughout the entire study period. Phosphate restriction was induced by the addition of dihydroxyaluminum amino acetate (a phosphate binder) to the diet of the phosphate-restricted group. At the conclusion of the study the survival rate was 66.67% in the restricted animals vs. 22.22% in the nonrestricted animals. Also, both the urine protein excretion and plasma creatinine levels were significantly less in the restricted group. From these studies it is difficult to conclude that dietary factors other than phosphate restriction are responsible for the prevention of renal functional deterioration in this experimental form of renal disease.

Other investigators have also confirmed this finding. Brown et al. studied the effect of phosphate restriction in another species, dogs, also with remnant kidneys. The one-year (morbidity) mortality in the dogs maintained on the low-phosphorus diet was 8.3% as compared with 66.7% in dogs maintained on a normal-phosphorus diet. Similarly, renal function at 1 year was twice as good in the surviving animals in the low-phosphorus group as in those on the normal-phosphorus diet. Recently, Harris has shown that phosphate restriction reduces proteinuria in uninephrectomized rats, rats with Adriamycin nephrotoxic reaction, and animals with experimentally induced diabetes mellitus. These various animal studies would suggest that dietary phosphorus restriction exerts a beneficial effect on a variety of types of experimental renal diseases in two separate animal species.

Human studies are much more difficult to interpret as regards a possible beneficial effect of phosphate or protein restriction on CRF. By far, the majority of studies in man have utilized a combination of dietary protein and phosphate restriction, which has made it impossible to determine which of these dietary constituents might be important in mediating any response noted. Even more important have been the flaws in the design of most human studies. Most investigators have assumed that the reciprocal of the plasma creatinine against time is represented in most patients as a straight line. However, in some series, up to 30% of the calculated slopes have been found to change with time. Another factor that has not been taken into consideration is the effect of protein restriction on creatinine formation. It has previously been shown that exogenously ingested creatine can account for as much as 15% of the plasma creatinine level. In addition, with a continuing protein restriction, a reduction in muscle mass as measured by a reduction in midarm muscle circumference has been noted. This in turn would result in a reduction in the endogenous production of creatinine. Both of these factors would falsely lower the plasma creatinine values and in turn alter the slope of the reciprocal of creatinine plotted against time. Because of this, it has been suggested that other means of estimating GFR should be used such as isotopic measurements or the determination of the combined measurement of creatinine and urea clearances. Possibly even more important is the placebo effect of clinical trials. Clinically, it has been well documented that even without any dietary manipulation the rate of renal function deterioration may be decreased providing there is intensive follow-up, increased frequency of visits, and better control of hypertension.

Only well-controlled studies that pay close attention to the measurement of GFR and the placebo effect will make it possible to determine what (if any) effect dietary manipulation can have on renal disease. With the dietary manipulations currently used, it may be impossible to determine whether any realized benefit is a result of phosphate or protein restriction or a combination of both.

In spite of the deficiencies noted above, the majority of studies reported would suggest that dietary restriction of protein might exert a beneficial effect for human renal disease. However, several other reports are not totally consistent with this contention. A recent study describes a number of patients with advanced renal failure maintained on a very-low-protein diet who had progression of renal failure. It was not until ketoacid analogues were substituted for the essential amino acid supplement that the progression of renal failure was slowed. This suggests that factors other than pure protein restriction may have played a more important role in reducing the rate of functional deterioration.

An additional study in humans showed that a combination of low-protein and low-phosphorus diet was much more effective in reducing the rate of renal functional deterioration than dietary protein restriction alone. This observation was based on the actual measurement of creatinine clearance rather than simply the determination of serum creatinine levels.

Although numerous animal studies have been used as additional support for the beneficial effect of dietary protein restriction on preservation of renal function, a number of them suffer from some deficiencies. Frequently, the protein-restricted diet has resulted in severe protein malnutrition in the animals. In addition, dietary controls have not usually been pair-fed, and in most studies (unlike some of the phosphate-restriction studies) there has been little attempt to control calorie intake or the inorganic constituents, including phosphate, of the diet. In almost all of the studies, protein restriction has been initiated either before or at the time of induction of renal failure. Therefore, it is less clear what effect protein restriction has on the course of renal failure after the disease has been well established.

Most studies supporting a beneficial effect of protein restriction have been performed in animals with the remnant kidney. Results reported in animals with experimental glomerulonephritis have been less consistent. In fact, a recent report would suggest that a high-protein diet actually improves renal function and survival in rats with nephrotoxic serum nephritis. The same study also found that a high-protein diet reduced tubulointerstitial disease.

Certainly, a strong argument can be made that protein restriction exerts a protective effect in the progression of renal disease by normalizing altered intrarenal hemodynamic events in the remnant kidney model. However, this argument is not so powerful or convincing in other models of renal failure. Little evidence exists that the hemodynamic changes found in the remnant kidney occur in experimental models of glomerulonephritis. Also, recent studies with the obese Zucker rat and spontaneously hypertensive rats with streptozocin-induced diabetes cast some doubt that altered intrarenal hemodynamics are important in the etiology of these renal diseases. Of course, one should not underestimate how significant systemic hypertension is in compounding the initial renal injury.

In summary, it would seem that at least under certain experimental conditions both dietary protein and phosphate restriction can exert a protective effect on some forms of experimental renal disease, preventing progressive functional deterioration. At this time it is much less convincing that either of these manipulations offers any benefit for humans with CRF.

In the animal studies there is increasing evidence that both protein and phosphate dietary restriction may exert protective effects by separate and distinct mechanisms. This evidence is based on the finding that glomerular and tubulointerstitial disease appear to result from different causes since these two processes can be separated by various dietary manipulations. At this time it would appear that glomerular injury, at least in some forms of experimental renal disease, is mediated by altered intrarenal hemodynamic events that can be modified by protein restriction. In contrast, tubulointerstitial injury is induced by other factors, possibly renal parenchymal calcification, which can be attenuated by phosphate restriction. It remains to be seen whether a combination of dietary protein and phosphate restriction may be operative in a synergistic fashion to retard progressive functional deterioration in a diseased kidney. Additional studies are obviously required before firm guidelines can be given for the dietary management of CRF in man.

Bibliography

1. Barsotti G, Giannoni A, Morelli E, et al: The decline of renal function slowed by very low phosphorus intake in chronic renal patients following a low nitrogen diet. *Clin Nephrol* 1984; 21:54–59.
2. Bucht H, Ahlberg M, Alvestrand A, et al: The effect of low protein diet on the progression of renal failure in man, in Bertani T, Remuzzi G, Garattini S (eds): *Drugs and Kidney*. New York, Raven Press, 1986, pp 257–267.
3. El Nahas AM, Kohls GA: Dietary treatment of chronic renal failure: Ten unanswered questions. *Lancet* 1986; 1:597–600.
4. El Nahas AM, Zoob SN, Evans DJ, et al: Chronic renal failure after nephrotoxic nephritis in rats: Contributions to progression. *Kidney Int* 1987; 32:173–180.

5. Laouari D, Kleinknecht C: The role of nutritional factors in the course of experimental renal failure. *Am J Kidney Dis* 1985; 3:147–156.
6. Lumlertgul D, Burke TJ, Gillum DM, et al: Phosphate depletion arrests progression of chronic renal failure independent of protein intake. *Kidney Int* 1986; 29:658–666.

Rebuttal: Affirmative
Thomas H. Hostetter, M.D., and Anthony C. Wooley, M.D.

It is less a matter of specific factual disagreement than one of perspective and emphasis that characterizes our criticism of Dr. Alfrey's position paper. As summarized in Figure 2, there is little question that a variety of nonhemodynamic factors unrelated to protein intake can contribute to progressive renal injury. A further exploration of such factors should continue to improve our understanding of mechanisms of renal injury and, one hopes, provide the basis for clinically useful treatments for patients with renal diseases. However, to suggest as Dr. Alfrey does that a variety of dietary manipulations can have protective effects in experimental renal diseases equal to those of protein restriction may be misleading or at least inadequately supported.

We suggest that the experimental and clinical literature on protein restriction in preventing progressive renal injury has at present provided a greater degree of scientific validation than other theories regarding dietary metabolic factors on the basis of three points. First, theories of dietary protein and its influence on renal function and renal disease have been studied in a large number of diverse setting in animals and humans, utilizing a broad range of experimental techniques. Second, there is much clinical evidence (albeit experimentally imperfect) suggesting that protein restriction in the absence of chronic malnutrition can exert a clinically important beneficial effect on the progression of a variety of human renal diseases. This evidence is adequately reviewed in our position paper (see Fig 1). Third, there are plausible and experimentally testable theories as to the mechanism by which dietary protein may influence renal injury.

The variety of experimental renal diseases in which protein restriction has resulted in attenuated injury, decreased proteinuria, or reduction of glomerular hypertension is impressive. In addition to the remnant kidney model, which represents a fairly pure form of progressive renal injury independent of any specific initiating mechanisms, experimental studies have demonstrated significant effects in experimental diabetic nephropathy, experimental lupus, models of experimental glomerulonephritis, and even models of experimental tubulointerstitial disease. Clinical studies have demonstrated beneficial effects of protein restriction in patients with glomerular and nonglomerular disease, in immunologically mediated and nonimmunologically mediated disease, and even in genetic renal disease such as adult polycystic kidney disease. These effects have been studied histologically, by measurement of GFR by various methods, by quantitation of proteinuria, by micropuncture measurements of glomerular function, and by a variety of other methods. The criticism that protein restriction in experimental disease has resulted in severe malnutrition is not valid for many protein studies and is perhaps a more valid criticism of the experimental studies of phosphorus depletion, which more often have resulted in progressive weight loss in experimental animals. In addition, the assertion that protein restriction may not have an important effect on the course of renal failure after renal disease is well established is contradicted by the human studies of protein restriction, which in many cases included patients with advanced renal failure. In addition, the findings of Nath et al.,[1] demonstrating that late intervention with dietary protein restriction in remnant kidney disease has a profound ameliorating effect on renal function histology and intrarenal hemodynamics, further make Dr. Alfrey's criticism puzzling.

By contrast, phosphorus restriction, particularly in the absence of chronic malnutrition (tested in a relatively small number of studies in a relatively small number of experimental settings), has been little studied in human renal diseases. The one available published study by Barrientos et al. failed to find any benefit to phosphate restriction. Data for an important role of lipids and other metabolic factors, though intriguing, are preliminary and have yet to be subjected to validation by multiple investigators and multiple methods, as has been done with protein restriction. Again, this is a matter of emphasis; we do not argue that there is not a role of dietary phosphorus or other dietary constituents in progressive renal injury but rather that the experimental evidence for these factors is not yet well established, and moreover clinical evidence is almost nonexistent.

Perhaps equally important is the compelling evidence that glomerular hyperperfusion and hyperfiltration play a prominent role in progressive renal injury. To reiterate points made in our position paper, glomerular hyperperfusion and hyperfiltration has been demonstrated in a wide variety of experimental renal diseases. Strong evidence for such hemodynamic changes can be adduced for human conditions of reduced renal mass, due to either chronic renal disease or uninephrectomy. The link between dietary protein and elevations in the renal blood flow, GFR, and glomerular capillary pressure are well established. In dogs, humans, or rats, a protein meal or amino acid infusion will result in a prompt increase in renal blood flow and GFR and chronic protein feeding will lead to sustained hyperfiltration and hyperperfusion. Conversely, both acute and chronic protein restriction, even to a degree that allows neutral nitrogen balance and preservation of normal nutritional parameters, will result in a reversal of these hemodynamic changes. That prevention of hyperfiltration and glomerular hypertension decreases renal injury is suggested not only by dietary protein restriction studies but also by the work of Anderson and coworkers.[2] Such studies have shown that the reversal of renal hemodynamic changes by converting enzyme inhibitors, a mechanism completely separate from that of protein restriction, can result in a similar dramatic prevention of renal injury. This effect has also been shown in experimental diabetes and suggested in short-term human studies as well.

Dr. Alfrey also suggests that although glomerular injury might be explained by hemodynamic injuries, other theories must be invoked to explain the tubulointerstitial injury seen in chronic renal diseases. A possible mechanism for tubulointerstitial injury is that of interstitial calcium phosphate deposition. This is the most widely cited theory explaining the effects of dietary phosphate restriction. However, another intriguing theory that might link dietary protein intake to tubulointerstitial injury is suggested by the work of Nath et al.[3] These authors demonstrated that elevated single-nephron ammonia production rates seen in chronic renal disease can stimulate the alternative pathway of complement by the nonenzymatic amidization of C3. Such injury was ameliorated by systemic alkalinization with bicarbonate. This theory could be linked to dietary protein intake in that dietary protein, and specifically sulfur-containing amino acids, constitute a major part of the daily acid load, and elevated single-nephron ammonia genesis would tend to elevate interstitial ammonia levels. Such theories all remain speculative and will undoubtedly undergo considerable modification in coming years. However, in some theories, linking protein intake glomerular hemodynamics and progressive renal injuries would seem to explain a greater variety of clinical and experimental observations and would seem to be supported by a broader variety of evidence than current competing theories. However, it should be noted that many of the proposed mechanisms are not mutually exclusive; indeed they may be synergistic, for example, hyperlipidemia and capillary hypertension.

In summary, although excess dietary protein intake is unlikely to be the whole explanation for progressive renal injury, its effect seems to be robust and reproducible and is supported by a compelling if incomplete theory of mechanism of injury. Such a theory does not exclude other important mediators of injury such as the role proposed for dietary phosphorus. The exposition of these factors and the unravelling of their interactions with renal hemodynamics and dietary protein is an enticing challenge for nephrology in coming years.

References

1. Nath KA, Kren SM, Hostetter TH: Dietary protein restriction in established renal injury in the rat. *JCI* 1986; 78:1199–1205.
2. Anderson S, Rennke H, Brenner BM: Therapeutic advantages of converting enzyme inhibitors in arresting renal disease associated with systemic hypertension in rats. *JCI* 1986; 77:1993.
3. Nath KA, Hostetter MK, Hostetter TH: The pathophysiology of chronic tubulointerstitial injury in rats. *JCI* 1985; 76:667.

Rebuttal: Negative
Allen C. Alfrey, M.D.

Ever since Farr and Smadel[1] first described the protective effect of a protein-restricted diet in nephrotoxic serum nephritis in 1939, there have been numerous studies regarding dietary protein restriction in experimental renal disease. Unfortunately, by far the majority of studies, including that of Farr and Smadel, have utilized protein calorie malnutrition rather than simply protein restriction. Essentially, all studies that have been shown to exert a beneficial effect in rats, including those referred to by Dr. Hostetter,[2] have used diets containing 6% to 7% protein. It is well recognized that rats maintained on this amount of protein restriction have marked malnutrition as exemplified by severe impairment of growth and weight gain. Moreover, if an attempt is made to supplement the 7% protein diet with only 1% amino acids, the preventive effect the restricted protein has on renal functional deterioration is largely lost.[3] This suggests that malnutrition may be more important than protein restriction in preventing functional deterioration. It has further been shown that a 14% protein diet, which is the minimum dietary protein in rats consistent with normal growth and weight gain, was much less efficacious in preventing functional deterioration than a 7% protein diet.[4] In fact, to show a benefit of higher-protein diets that do not cause malnutrition, comparisons have frequently been made with animals maintained on a super normal protein intake. Strangely enough, however, it has also been found that under certain conditions a high-protein diet may also be protective of renal functional deterioration, again possibly as a result of reduced food intake.

Another major problem with most protein-restriction studies has been the fact that other dietary constituents have not been controlled. Even in Hostetter's study,[2] where other dietary constituents in the control diet were matched to the low-protein diet, the animals were not pair-fed; there is reason to doubt that the amount the control group ingested was the same as in the protein-restricted group. Measurement of dietary intake at one point in time when animals were placed in metabolic cages may not reflect intake in animals maintained under different conditions over several months' duration. With the majority of these studies, one could infer that malnutrition was as significant a factor in protection from renal functional deterioration as was protein restriction.

As pointed out by El Nahas and Kohls,[5] the majority of human studies purporting to show a beneficial effect of protein restriction on CRF have some glaring deficiencies. According to these investigators, the major problems of protein restriction studies concern lack of controls in all but one study, inappropriate means of assessing renal failure, and failure to account for the placebo effect. Nahas and Kohls indicated that decreased dietary protein and creatine intake with a consequent loss of muscle mass could significantly reduce creatinine production. This reduction could have a major effect on using the reciprocal of the creatinine plotted against time as an index of change in rate of functional deterioration.

A point of equal concern is the so-called placebo effect. It has been well documented by Bucht et al.[6] that patients having more frequent follow-up with better control of blood pressure and other factors can have marked improvement in the rate of functional deterioration without any dietary manipulation. These authors conclude that only prospective, randomized studies controlled for the increased frequency and quality of care can clearly show whether protein restriction has any beneficial effect on preserving renal function in patients with CRF. Until such controlled studies have been carried out, prescribing low-protein diets for patients with CRF seems unwarranted, especially considering the danger, expense, and inconvenience of such diets.

References

1. Farr LE, Smadel JE: The effect of dietary protein on the course of nephrotoxic nephritis in rats. *J Experimental Med* 1939; 70:615–622.
2. Hostetter TH: Dietary protein and the progression of renal disease. In press.
3. Laouari M, Kleinknecht C: The role of nutritional factors in the course of experimental renal disease. *Am J Kidney Dis* 1985; 3:147–156.
4. Kleinknecht C, Salusky I, Broyer M, et al: Effect of various protein diets on growth, renal function, and survival of uremic rats. *Kidney Int* 1979; 15:534–541.
5. El Nahas AM, Kohls GA: Dietary treatment of chronic renal failure: Ten unanswered questions. *Lancet* 1986; 1:597–600.
6. Bucht H, Ahlberg M, Alvestrand A, et al: The effect of low protein diet on the progression of renal failure in man, in Bertani T, Remuzzi G, Garattini S (eds): *Drugs and Kidney*. New York, Raven Press, 1986, pp 257–267.

Editor's Comments
H. Verdain Barnes, M.D.

Chronic renal failure appears to have at least three or four stages, ranging from a diminution in renal reserve to frank uremia. The early clinical manifestations of this progressive disease process may go unnoticed by the patient, or he or she may attribute the symptoms to other causes. Consequently, it is virtually impossible to know how many in our population might benefit from a method of forestalling or preventing the natural progression of CRF to a point where dialysis or a new kidney are the only options to preserve life. Since it is estimated that over 60,000 die each year of a renal or genitourinary disorder, the number who might benefit appears to be substantial. In this context, this debate on restricting protein or phosphate intake as a method of retarding the progression of CRF is of particular interest and importance to the clinician. Since the renal physiology and natural history of chronic renal disease are both complex and are influenced by the individual's own biogenetic characteristics, it is not surprising that the debate is vigorous by these scholars of renal disease.

Our authors, Drs. Hostetter and Wooley on the side of dietary protein restriction and Dr. Alfrey on the side of dietary phosphate restriction, seem to agree on some issues. They agree that (1) the natural history of CRF is one of progression over time, though they do not agree as to how this can be most accurately documented; (2) definitive clinical conclusions cannot be drawn from currently available animal or human studies, although each has logical arguments supporting the importance of their intervention; (3) both protein and phosphate restriction may play a role, possibly by a different mechanism, and that they may be additive or synergistic in effect; and (4) continued study in this important area is mandated. With these points I also agree. However, I am skeptical that a definitive clinical answer is likely to be forthcoming from human studies due to the individual variations in the rate of progression of CRF and the individual responses to therapy, including the elusive placebo effect. On the other hand, additional supportive evidence regarding their effectiveness as well as their potential additive or synergistic effect would be of use to the clinician caring for patients with CRF.

The animal studies cited by these authors provide an important background and theory for the development of human studies, as well as the pathogenesis of CRF, but suffer in this setting as in others by not necessarily having direct correlation to the human response to a disease process or to a therapeutic intervention. Dr. Alfrey's point about the need to use pair-fed animals in the protein-restriction studies is, I believe, well taken. On the other side, Drs. Hostetter and Wooley make a good point concerning Dr. Alfrey's statement regarding protein restriction being of little or no proved potential benefit in well-established CRF.

246

Currently, more data are available from human studies regarding protein than phosphate restriction, but these data, though clearly suggesting a benefit, have in my opinion not been unequivocally documented. Nonetheless, the restriction of dietary protein or phosphate or both seems to me to be reasonable in adults with CRF, even though the potential benefits of long-term restriction of these two important nutrients or the potential longitudinal effects of restriction on other aspects of the health and function of muscle, bone, and other systems, as well as healing, are unknown. In children and adolescents with CRF, the restriction of protein is fraught with a clear potential for growth retardation and an ultimate compromise of adult stature. The restriction of phosphate is also a potential hazard in this age group. Based on available data, it may be prudent at this time to avoid the use of a major phosphate or protein restriction in these patients until they complete their growth and development. If either is restricted, I believe, it should be done with caution, with careful and frequent assessments of growth (every 4 to 6 months). Although not directly addressed in this debate, our growing knowledge of renal prostaglandin synthesis and action may offer an additional approach for delaying or perhaps preventing for some period the relentless longitudinal progression of CRF.[1] As I view it, the search for an effective intervention is just beginning and should be vigorously pursued.

Reference

1. Epstein M (ed): Proceedings of a Symposium. Prostaglandins and the Kidney. *Am J Med* 1986; 80(suppl 1A).

Patient Autonomy Eliminates a Role for Paternalism in the Doctor-Patient Relationship

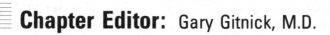

Chapter Editor: Gary Gitnick, M.D.

Affirmative: Angela R. Holder, LL.M.
Counsel for Medicolegal Affairs, Yale
University School of Medicine and Yale-New
Haven Hospital; Clinical Professor of
Pediatrics (Law), Yale University School of
Medicine, New Haven, Connecticut

Negative: Thomas P. Duffy, M.D.
Professor of Medicine, Section of
Hematology, Department of Internal
Medicine, Yale University School of
Medicine, New Haven, Connecticut

Debates in Medicine 1:248–268, 1988
© 1988, Year Book Medical Publishers, Inc.
0887-218X/88/01-248-268-$04.00

Affirmative

Angela R. Holder, LL.M.

Webster's New International Dictionary defines autonomy as "the quality or state of being independent, free and self-directing: individual or group freedom . . . . the sovereignty of reason in the sphere of morals: possession of moral freedom or self-determination . . . independence from the organism as a whole in the capacity of a part for growth, reactivity or responsiveness." Paternalism is defined as "the care or control of subordinates in a fatherly manner."

Paternalism is just not what it used to be. If Clarence Day (of *Life With Father*) or Frank Gilbreth *(Cheaper by the Dozen)* were to return in 1987, they would be disconcerted to discover that God-fearing, self-respecting men can't even be paternalistic in their own houses anymore, much less anywhere else. Mrs. Day would be likely to work on Wall Street and Mrs. Gilbreth would be a professor of engineering. If they were lucky, their teenage daughters would be clients at Planned Parenthood and the courts would tell them there is nothing they can do about either. To the anguish of the extreme conservative who thinks the American family has degenerated into immorality, old-fashioned paternalism is out of style. Real men may or may not eat quiche, but most of them know how to cook.

Grover Cleveland said in his Inaugural Address in 1893, "The lessons of paternalism ought to be unlearned," and it seems that for those who would like to recreate the authority of old-time paternalism, things have been going downhill ever since.

There are no William Henry Vanderbilts thundering "the public be damned" nowadays; their granddaughters run jeans empires that succeed because the public wants to buy the product; those who work on Wall Street in the tradition begun by the Vanderbilts and Morgans are going to jail for insider trading violations. Fathers change diapers instead of issuing orders.

Changes in society, both within the family and in the individual's relationship with others in his or her community, reflect an entirely different view of authority from that acceptable 50 years ago. These changes are, of course, reflected in the relationships between physicians and their patients, but there is nothing unique about that. At the time the AMA's first Code of Ethics was written in 1847 indicating that patients' "obedience . . . should be prompt and explicit,"[1] there were also no laws prohibiting child abuse, since any such legislation would have infringed on a father's right to do as he pleased with his children.

Fatherhood, without the fire and brimstone, and the practice of medicine, without demands to patients for polite and unquestioning obedience, are both flourishing. Daddies still won't let little kids run out into the street, and a trip to the doctor for a prescription for hypertension medication still isn't like going to the supermarket and picking one detergent instead of another.

When courts began to talk about informed consent as the doctrine exists today, the social context in which they operated had begun to be quite different from the authoritarian society in which we had lived. The first decision in which the term was used, *Salgo v Leland Stanford University Board of Trustees,*[2] was handed down by the California Supreme Court in 1957, the same year President Eisenhower sent troops to Little Rock, Arkansas, so that black children could go to an integrated high school as ordered by the federal court. I do not think this was coincidence; I see both actions as resulting from the same social forces. Long-standing acceptance of patterns of authority was beginning to dissipate. People in American society were beginning to question the validity of decisions made about their lives by those in authority, who, among other things, did not live with the pain of the consequences.

What, after all, is informed consent about? The most succinct description I have ever seen comes from a 1973 decision of the Ohio Supreme Court[3]:

[T]he informed consent doctrine is based on the proposition that every competent person is the final arbiter of whether or not he gets cut, by whom he gets cut, and where he gets cut. A patient has the sovereign choice of whether he will submit to surgery in the course of the diagnosis and treatment and in order to make this choice meaningful and realistic the doctor is under a legal duty to disclose to a patient any serious risks involved in the contemplated surgery and the alternatives available to him, including the risks of nontreatment.

Understanding what one is getting into and making choices about it within the framework of a given set of circumstances is all that respect for patient autonomy requires.

Unlike the other authors in this book, I view the physician-patient relationship from the perspective of a patient. Some of the physician readers will have, at some time in their careers, gotten a divorce, been sued for malpractice, or had their income tax returns audited. In these cases, I assume you consulted a lawyer, which is what I am.

I assume that you were as frightened and unnerved by your legal problem as I am when I think I am sick. When you went to your lawyer, I doubt seriously that after you explained the problem you were handed the Internal Revenue Code or textbooks on domestic relations or malpractice and told to go decide what you wanted to do and come back when you'd made up your mind. If your autonomy were the single value in your relationship with your lawyer, that might very well have happened. You would have come to him or her to be "free and self-directing."

However, what I would hope any lawyer would have done is to begin by asking you to explain everything you know about the problem and then telling you what he or she thinks the legal situation is likely to be. After several further visits and exchanges of more information, you would consider your options—in the case of the malpractice suit, to settle or to go to trial, with attendant publicity and a chance of either winning and being vindicated or losing and having a large judgment levied against you. What you eventually decided to do would probably be based not only on what the lawyer told you but would also reflect your general approach to risks in your life, a factor that your lawyer can't possibly know about you. Some people are gamblers, some people are risk-aversive. In any case, you would not want to tell your lawyer what the facts had been and that you didn't think you had made any mistakes and have him or her say, "Well, of course we must settle the case at once," indicate that there is no need for further discussion, and say that the next client is waiting. If, to open the interview, the first thing the lawyer had said to you was "Hi, Charlie, I'm Mr. Jones," you would have felt most demoralized by the whole experience.

It is likely that the last time you saw your lawyer, your autonomy was respected, your stated goals were considered, and decisions were made in an ongoing dialogue between you and your counsel. In short, you gave informed consent in a situation in which you are as uncomfortable as your patients are when they come to see you. I, the patient, am just as confused and frightened in your office as you, the client, are in mine. We each come for help and we come to someone we believe knows more about solving our problem than we do.

Autonomy

How, then, do we define autonomy as it becomes relevant to such a relationship as that between a physician and patient or a lawyer and client? If I decide that I wish to buy a new skirt, first I decide how much, approximately, I can afford to spend and then I go shopping. How many stores I visit depends on the degree of my desire to spend my time at this endeavor instead of doing something else, my energy level at the time, my patience (or lack thereof), and whether or not my feet hurt. What sort of skirt I buy depends on what is available within the stores I have decided to visit, what within that stock is appropriate for the occasions for which I am buying the skirt, how well it fits into the general wardrobe of skirts I already own, and what I like and what I don't within that subset. When I finally find a skirt I wish to buy and leave the store with it, I have made a classically autonomous decision. All by myself I have demonstrated the Beauchamp and Childress[4] definition of autonomy: "Autonomy is a form of personal liberty of action where the individual determines his or her own course of action in accordance with a plan chosen by himself or herself. . . . A person's autonomy is his or her independence, self-reliance and self-contained ability to decide."

The reason that there has been perennial conflict in discussions of the physician-patient relationship between autonomy and paternalism is that the skirt-buying model of autonomy, usually presented by those who wish to argue in favor of paternalism, is inapplicable in any context involving a fiduciary relationship. A fiduciary relationship is one in which a person, with superior knowledge of some subject matter, has a duty, created by his undertaking, to act primarily for another's benefit.[5] The fiduciary relationship is founded on trust and confidence reposed by one person in the integrity and fidelity, as well as the superior knowledge, of another.[6] Physicians are fiduciaries of their patients, lawyers of their clients, guardians of their wards, and trustees of their beneficiaries. The fiduciary obligation is based on an affirmative duty to disclose all relevant information to the beneficiary. "Caveat emptor" has no place in any fiduciary situation. The notion of this sort of special relationship and its concomitant obligations of disclosure evolved from the law of trusts. The earliest example I can find of a formal trust occurred in the year 1225, some centuries before courts began writing opinions about informed consent, but the basic obligations are just the same.[7]

What are the real differences between my autonomy when I buy a skirt and my autonomy when I visit my physician or yours when you visit your lawyer? There are several. One is that I know or can find out anything I want to know about skirts without having to ask advice. Second, I am presumably not nervous or frightened about the consequences of buying a skirt. Thus, though there are psychological determinants of my deciding to buy a skirt in the first place and the reason I select the one I buy in the second, it is largely an intellectual decision unrelated to emotional trauma. If, however, I don't feel well and I make an appointment with my physician, I do so because I want help and he or she knows more about what will help than I do. What I seek is advice, not a product. I may also be extremely upset and frightened and I wish to have that fear treated with respect. Therefore, to discuss autonomy in the context of relationships between physicians and patients or lawyers and clients by using the definition applicable to buying skirts is to mix apples and oranges and wonder why the apple pie tastes like marmalade.

My autonomy as a patient—and yours as the client of a lawyer—is best served if the professional adopts the Kantian principle of respect for persons. "So act as to treat humanity, whether in thine own person or in that of any other, in every case as an end withal, never as a means only."[8] That means that my desire for autonomy—to make decisions about my body—should include an understanding that, in addition to my intellect, my physician must factor into our discussion my emotions, my simple lack of knowledge about the subject of the conversation (in the situation in which I am intelligent enough to understand information provided to me, but I just don't happen to know it), and my immediate capacity to absorb the information provided if I have just had very bad news or am feeling so ill that I am not paying attention. Discussion may require several meetings and repetition. Only then can I possibly choose among my alternatives or decide that I just want to be left alone. There is a little informing and a little consenting,[9] another bit of informing and another bit of consenting, and eventually we arrive at an understanding of what my physician and I agree to do, whether it is that he will treat my problem and by what means or that I will decide that I want to be left alone. Not until I have the necessary information, however, and am able to process it correctly am I operating as an autonomous person.

As Jay Katz[1] has written:

Decision making in medicine, in order to safeguard the autonomy of both parties, must become a joint undertaking that depends more on the nature and quality of the entire give-and-take process than on whether a particular disclosure has or has not been made. Translating the ingredients of this into useful legal and medical prescriptions that respect patients' wishes to maintain and surrender autonomy, as well as physicians' unending struggles with omnipotence and impotence in the light of medical uncertainty is a difficult task and has not been pursued in any depth.

So a patient's or a client's autonomy is a process. As I understand more about why my stomach hurts and you, in my office, understand more about what will happen in the malpractice suit against you, both you and I are becoming autonomous and eventually will be able to make our choices about future actions or inactions.

Paternalism

Having established, I hope, that autonomy in the context of a fiduciary relationship of any sort is not the same thing as autonomy in other areas, we must next examine paternalism in the same context.

Hans Jonas,[10] writing about "the right to die," has said:

For myself, I venture this statement of principle: ultimately the patient's autonomy should be honored, that is, not be prevented by deception from making its best-informed supreme choice unless he wants to be deceived. To find this out is part of the true physician's competence, not learned in medical school. He has to size up the person—no mean feat of intuition. Satisfied that the patient really wants the truth—his mere saying so is not proof enough—the physician is morally and contractually bound to give it to him. . . Otherwise, and especially if there is a choice to be made, the mature subject's right to full disclosure, earnestly claimed and convincingly apparent as his will, ought to have its way in extremis, overruling mercy and whatever custodial authority a doctor may have on behalf of the patient's presumed good.

The sort of medical paternalism that, for example, resulted in a woman with breast cancer never being told about modified radical mastectomies or lumpectomies with radiation, because her surgeon thought that a radical mastectomy was the only acceptable method of treatment, has gone, in theory if not in practice. In researching this chapter, I could not find a current reference to support that approach to patient care.

As Clarence Day would find *Life With Father* quite different in the 1980s from the authoritarianism of his era, so, too, has medicine changed. It may be that some benefit, however minimal, has come from "the malpractice crisis," because whatever physicians may actually believe about the capacity of patients to understand what they are told and the capacity of patients to make intelligent choices, they at least know that if they do not disclose alternatives, they may be sued successfully for failure to obtain informed consent.

If one equates paternalism with the old-time method of fatherhood, people nowadays talk to their children, too. The choice a 2-year-old may make on a given morning is whether he wants to wear his red sweater or his blue sweater to nursery school. He is not asked whether he wants to wear a sweater, but he has made a choice and he will grow up making choices. Children are heard as well as seen. "Do it because I told you to" is now more likely to be a statement of parental exasperation than it is to be a considered approach to child-rearing. People are growing up accustomed to making choices and when they walk into a physician's office they do not abandon their skills at living their lives and protecting their own interests. Whether medicine has chosen to abandon its posture of "doctor knows best" or whether patients have simply refused to put up with it and voted with their feet for physicians who treat them as intelligent beings, times have changed. The paterfamilias would not only get laughed out of the living room at home, he would lose patients at the office.

The ideal relationship between physician and patient or lawyer and client is rarely realized in practice. Paternalism takes less time than dialogue. Some patients and clients are too frightened or too unintelligent ever to understand what the physician or lawyer is trying to tell them. Some physicians are unable to explain medical procedures in terms intelligible to their lawyers, much less their patients, and some lawyers are just as incomprehensible. Under DRGs and other cost-containment mechanisms, the thing physicians do that is least compensated is to talk to patients, and that doubtless has an effect on the time the physician is able to devote to such discussions. So paternalism still occurs in both law and medicine; patient or client autonomy still may or may not exist in any given case. However, that is now the ideal that is taught and toward which medicine seems to be willing to strive.

Conclusion

Thus, if I were to define autonomy by the skirt-buying model, it is clear that the answer I would give in this debate is affirmative. Patient autonomy does eliminate old-fashioned paternalism. What the question ignores, however, is that that is not the model for physician-patient interactions. The autonomy of a patient is not unlike the autonomy of a student. Once the basic lesson is learned, the wise teacher allows the student to choose the ways in which the knowledge is applied, thus affirming the student's autonomy and preparing him or her for independent work at the next level. Perhaps the role of paternalism in medicine in the future will become that of a physician who thinks of a dialogue with patients as a teacher thinks of explaining a new concept to students. I certainly want that for myself in my capacity as a patient. I do not want to choose medications as I choose detergents at the supermarket. I go to the physician for advice and help as well as for information, and receiving it does not violate my autonomy as long as I am free to accept it, reject it, or go for another opinion to help me make up my mind.

References

1. Katz J: *The Silent World of Doctor and Patient.* New York, Free Press, 1984, pp 21, 84.
2. *Salgo v Leland Stanford University Board of Trustees,* 317 P2d 170 (Cal 1957).
3. *Congreve v Holmes,* 308 NE2d 765 (Ohio 1973).
4. Beauchamp T, Childress J: *Principles of Biomedical Ethics.* New York, Oxford University Press, 1979, pp 56–57.
5. *Haluka v Baker,* 66 Ohio App 308, 34 NE 2d 68, 1941.
6. *Kerrigan v O'Meara,* 71 Mont 1, 227 Pac 819, 821, 1926.
7. Holder AR: Do researchers and subjects have a fiduciary relationship? *IRB: Rev Hum Subjects Res* 1982; 4:6–7.
8. Lebacqz KA, Levine RJ: Respect for persons and informed consent to participate in research. *Clin Res* 1977; 25:101.
9. Levine RJ: *Ethics and Regulation of Clinical Research,* ed 2. Baltimore, Urban & Schwarzenberg, 1986, p 128.
10. Jonas H: The right to die. *Hastings Cent Rep* 1978; 4:33–34.

Negative
Thomas P. Duffy, M.D.

Few physicians, in their professional or private lives, are now so oblivious to the general public's disenchantment with authority that they would assume an absolute paternalistic stance in the doctor-patient relationship (DPR). Informed consent, patient autonomy, and patient will dominate this encounter, and ethicists and lawyers applaud this tilt or total shift in decision-making power in the sickroom. Some perceive physicians as neutral sources of information who assist patients in making their choices from a menu of medical care. The Hippocratic code of "do no harm" is of secondary importance to the supremacy of self-determination in medical decisions. Outcome of treatment has become less important than the patient's control of treatment. In this ill-advised pursuit of total autonomy, the patient may be depriving himself of his most valuable ally during illness, making a choice that has its misguided origins in a misinterpretation of the libertarian ethic and has implications for the DPR that may significantly alter the successful outcome of therapy.

The autonomy–patient rights model has its philosophical roots in the works of Mill[1] and Kant.[2] The primacy of autonomy in their teaching is based on the belief that autonomy is the ground of the dignity of human nature and of every rational nature; it is a prerequisite for all other virtues. Paternalism, acting on behalf of patients for their benefit but without their permission,[3] transgresses the patients' autonomy and is considered incompatible with Mill's dictum that "over himself, over his own body and mind, the individual is sovereign." Beneficence (doing good unto others) and nonmalfeasance (do no harm), the traditional underpinnings of the medical profession, have lost their preeminence in the DPR on the grounds that "the ability to choose is a good that is independent of the wisdom of what is chosen." But the attribution of total decision-making power to the patient may represent an exaggeration of Mill's conceptualization of rights and a failure to consider the altered status of the sick patient.

Mill excluded one act from his universal prohibition against paternalistic acts; this is the act of a man selling himself into slavery. In doing so, the man abdicates his liberty and forgoes any future use of it beyond that single act. But one possible outcome of total decision-making by the patient may be a fatal one, a decision to die because the immediate threat of suffering overshadows any promise of cure. The autonomous patient may decide to withdraw from treatment because sickness has distorted his outlook and he has never before witnessed the trajectory of illness. In declining appropriate treatment, the patient does not sell himself into slavery or abdicate his liberty but he may be abdicating his life. Libertarians might trumpet this choice as validating the importance of autonomy (freedom chosen over life), although common sense would suggest otherwise. For any physician participating in an unnecessary and improper choice of medical care by a patient, especially in circumstances that include a risk of death, the dilemma of beneficence vs. autonomy is usually decided in favor of beneficence. Mill did not think that society should tolerate a man's choice of slavery; most physicians do not think that a patient's autonomous but erroneous choice in medical care should necessarily be respected. The pleadings, legal maneuverings, and apprehension that surround the care of the Jehovah's Witness patient who refuses blood transfusions is a dramatic example of the physician stance regarding this issue; more subtle but no less difficult confrontations are commonplace in critical care units. The unnecessary prolongation of life by physicians is an appropriate target of criticism and intolerable from everyone's perspective. The unwise and inappropriate choice of premature death is just as intolerable from the physician's point of view.

Mill permitted a paternalistic stance to avoid a man's loss of liberty in choosing slavery; he also restricted the autonomous stance to "human beings in the maturity of their faculties." Children and retarded adults were considered still to require being taken care of by others and still to need protection against their own actions. It is in this respect that many advocates of paternalism find the defense of their cause.[4] With the onset of illness, the patient assumes a sick role with loss of autonomy. Restoration of health represents the return of autonomy. The doctor and patient are in a partnership to restore health and autonomy. The latter is not there to function as the primary determinant in the DPR. In this scenario, physician beneficence is viewed as the fount of autonomy and not as its destroyer.[5]

Any depiction of patients as children is obviously an unflattering one, and such a posture by physicians vis-à-vis patients would be cited as additional evidence of physician arrogance. But there is such a regression that sometimes accompanies illness; emotional disorders may hamper the optimal functioning of the body, and physical disorders may take a comparable toll of emotional resources. Anna Freud has written that every adult who is ill, who has a fever, who is in pain, or who expects an operation, returns to childhood in some way.[6] For children, parental paternalism is acceptable because it represents a future-oriented consent, a wager by the parent on the child's subsequent recognition of the wisdom of the choice or restriction. Is it so inappropriate and unacceptable to permit the physician to make such wagers when the alternative may be a bad medical outcome? Is the choice of what is to be done the exclusive privilege of the sick patient? When one is considering future-oriented consent, death would be a macabre termination of that trust. Parental paternalism is justified because it provides a wider range of freedom to the individual in question. It appears justifiable to consider that some medical paternalistic decisions also provide a like expansion of freedom when proper therapy conquers illness.

This justification does not apply to the situations that the critics of paternalism so rightly deride in the DPR. Unilateral decision-making without adequate conversation with patients is a condemnable misuse of the physician's power. The example of such abuse that is cited most frequently by ethicists opposed to paternalism is the surgical procedure of radical mastectomy used for treatment of breast malignancies.[7] The operation is now perceived as an aggressive assault on a woman's body in a mistaken surgical attempt to cure the disease. The recognition that breast cancer is frequently a systemic disorder because it is already disseminated at presentation was unknown until recently. Such knowledge required proof that some physicians were slow to learn and to believe. With the shift in the understanding of the disease, there was an alteration and expansion in the therapeutic options. Breast cancer became a "multispecialty" illness, with surgeons, radiotherapists, and oncologists collaborating in the therapies for this malignancy. Because there is no specific cure for breast cancer, optimal management now includes patient choice of the multiple modalities available. If and when a curative therapy becomes available, the forcefulness with which a specific therapy is offered will shift.

The critics of paternalism continue to cite the imbroglio of breast cancer management as a major example of paternalism in medicine. Removal of a woman's breast is frequently cited as the most egregious example of such behavior. Unfortunately, it is a better example of ignorance in medicine, of lack of knowledge, than it is of paternalism. No one is critical of amputation of an extremity to stay the threat of advancing gangrene. No physician chooses to mutilate a human body unless this is the only means of saving a life. Radical mastectomy was performed with this purpose in mind. With the growth in knowledge regarding other therapeutic options, the stance of medicine, formerly perceived as paternalistic, has changed in this setting. To continue to downplay beneficence because ignorance is confused with paternalism is a loss to both parties in the DPR.

An additional contribution to this controversy is the mishandling of experimental subjects by physicians.[8] Numerous examples of physician culpability in ignoring patient rights and informed consent in experiments fuel the ire that paternalism ignites in ethicists. But in entering an experimental trial, the patient is not participating in a DPR; in fact, the patient has become an experimental subject and the physician is functioning as a scientist. The appropriate outrage over transgressions in this setting should be directed against the proper target. This is the physician, not as a doctor but as a scientist, experimenting in quest of new knowledge. This ostensibly higher goal has unfortunately led some physicians to sacrifice not only patient autonomy but even beneficence in handling experimental subjects. This is the reason human investigation committees are so rigorous in protecting human subjects who participate in experimental protocols: such subjects are being used as means to the ends of scientific progress. Because of the difficult issues involved, many ethicists would prohibit any doctor from employing his own patients in his own experimental protocols. The leap from patient manipulation in a research setting to paternalistic manipulation in the DPR is untenable and should be exposed as fallacious in content. The DPR is not an extension of an experimental protocol.

But the brouhaha over physician mismanagement of breast malignancies or the manipulation or misuse of experimental subjects seems small when one considers the subtle, but real, alteration in the DPR that has evolved in the climate of absolute patient autonomy. Where beneficence is not greeted with disdain, the physician attends to the patient's needs in distress; the physician is not simply explaining or teaching patients about the available choices. In creating an atmosphere where the physician is only a conveyer of information, the physician may feel justified in functioning purely as a conduit of knowledge. Gone will be the important nerve to act on clinical intuition and the willingness to sustain a patient through a crisis for chances of a future cure; gone will be the traditional responsibility and altruism of the profession. An invaluable ally may be lost because the physician will feel justified in restricting the bounty of the encounter. The strident demands of autonomy could vitiate the important attending role of the profession.

Full patient autonomy unleashes another threat in medical care. In assuming greater responsibility for decision-making, the patient may miscalculate his command of the situation; the simple reflex of contacting the doctor may no longer be in place for the autonomous patient. Confronting the doctor could become threatening because the autonomous patient may perceive this as evidence of dependency. The valuable services of the physician would be sacrificed because the patient is unaware of the limits of his knowledge. In the strict adherence to a philosophical concept of rights and autonomy, the clinical outcome may be ignored—a Pyrrhic victory at best in the controversy between the ethicist and physician.

Any battle has its offensive and defensive components. The arguments in support of some paternalism in the DPR have been defensive up to this point. Clements and Sider[9] have mounted a different form of attack to repulse "medical ethics' assault upon medical values." They believe that the patient autonomy–rights model subverts values intrinsic to medicine, is without proven merit, and has attempted to replace the historical medical value system with an ill-fitting alternative. The autonomy is not grounded in the reality of clinical medicine and does not realistically address the complicated process of caring for the sick. It is as if no clearly defined solutions to clinical problems exist that transcend any argument regarding patient rights—no insulin for diabetes, penicillin for pneumococcal pneumonia, appendectomy for appendicitis. For a physician to accede to a patient's demand not be treated for such conditions would be a dereliction of physician responsibility.

Physicians are trained to recognize medical norms, and ethical treatment consists of trying to accomplish those norms. In circumstances where the norms are not established (breast cancer with its choice of mastectomy and/or chemotherapy and/or radiation therapy), the patient is obviously the individual who decides among the options with appropriate counsel from the physician. Where care is grounded in a scientific knowledge of the problem, patient preference is not a reliable basis for medical practice. There are shared medical views that constitute the basis of good medical care; to substitute autonomy for the goal of a good outcome is to belittle the contribution of medicine to patient care.

The primacy of patient autonomy in the DPR was stated to have its origins in the ethical teachings of Mill and Kant. Defense of a moral principle in the latter's canon depends on its being universally valid for everyone. It is strange that autonomy, defended on the basis of the categorical imperative wherein a maxim must be universalizable, is a restricted option in the different medical systems throughout the world. In Britain, medical care cannot have autonomy as a central tenet because of limitations in patient access to medical care; autonomy may exist over a limited range in this setting, although paternalistic direction of patient care is the likely outcome. Oriental societies perceive paternalism as the most acceptable mode of the DPR; the benificent physician may even *tell it like it isn't* if dealing with threatening medical information.[10] With the progressive bureaucratization of medicine, autonomy may not be an option even in the United States, where decision-making may no longer be in the hands of the physician. Such cultural relativism makes it questionable that autonomy is the overriding concern of the DPR. Rather, the overriding concern of physicians in all cultures is to return the sick to good health and to alleviate suffering. The focus on autonomy appears *myopic*.

Any attempt at imposing strict boundaries on decision-making in the DPR is futile because it ignores the reality of clinical medical practice. Most patients do not fearlessly brandish their expertise and decision-making powers at the height of illness, and no physician should purposely deceive his patients, even for their own good. Deceit would destroy the trust that graces the DPR, a partnership where shifts in decision-making ability are recognized and incorporated into the relationship. Some patients need to maintain a stronger posture of control and authority, whereas other patients delegate major decision-making responsibilities to their physicians. The fashion whereby these adjustments are made constitutes the art of medicine, with the wise physician recognizing the uniqueness of each encounter and modulating his intervention accordingly. The therapeutic ratio of autonomy to paternalism will differ for each patient and even for the same patient at different stages of an illness. At the height of illness, when emotional and physical resources are low, a more paternalistic intervention may be appropriate. As illness recedes, the patient becomes capable of greater autonomy in the partnership.

The controversy regarding patient autonomy and physician paternalism is therefore not to be solved by allusions to Mill or Kant or even the Hippocratic oath. Allegations of cultural relativism or minimalist ethics will also not resolve the debate.[11] Clements and Sider are correct in positioning the central role of shared medical knowledge and clinical norms in determining the outcome of the DPR; without these norms the DPR is an empty exercise in manners, better carried out in the drawing room than the clinic. This center of scientific acumen is surrounded by the richly textured art of medicine, which determines how that knowledge is dispensed. A beneficent outcome is the purpose for which the art and science of medicine is intended; the varying ingredients of autonomy and paternalism, whatever their mix, are only the seasonings of the main course. Physicians should not subvert or sacrifice good medical care for the process of decision-making. Rather, decision-making in the partnership should aid in realizing the proper end of medicine.

References

1. Mill JS: *On Liberty,* Hummelfarb G (ed). Harmondsworth, England, Penguin Books, 1974.
2. Kant I: *Groundwork of the Metaphysics of Morals,* Paton HJ (trans). New York, Harper & Row, 1964.
3. O'Neill O: Paternalism and partial autonomy. *J Med Ethics* 1984; 10:173–178.
4. Schoeman F: Parental discretion and children's rights: Background and implications for medical decision-making. *J Med Philos* 1985; 10:45–61.
5. Cassell E: The function of medicine. *Hastings Cent Rep* 1977; 7:16–19.
6. Freud A: The doctor-patient relationship, in Katz J (ed): Experimentation with human beings. New York, Russell Sage Foundation, 1972, pp 642–643.
7. Katz J: *The Silent World of Doctor and Patient.* New York, Macmillan Publishing Co, 1984.
8. Katz J: The regulation of human experimentation in the United States: A personal odyssey. *International Review Board* 1987; 9:1–6.
9. Clements C, Sider R: Medical ethics' assault upon medical values. *JAMA* 1983; 250:2011–2015.
10. Schor JD: "Wabi-Sabi." *JAMA* 1984; 252:3173.
11. Callahan D: Autonomy: A moral good, not a moral obsession. *Hastings Cent Rep* 1984; 14:40–42.

Rebuttal: Affirmative
Angela R. Holder, LL.M.

Contemporary writers in the field of medical law and ethics discuss autonomy, as did Mill and Kant, as a concept, but discussion of an idea in the abstract does not equate with the assumption that it will be translated literally into practice. To accept Dr. Duffy's version of the "total shift in decision-making power in the sickroom" is to assume that the person who is the patient wishes to relate to his or her physician in the same way he or she relates to the salesclerk asked to show all the different models of VCRs in the store. Dr. Duffy writes that "lawyers applaud this . . . total shift." I don't and I don't know any lawyers who do, in literal terms.

Absolute autonomy, like Aristotle's concept of absolute justice, cannot be attained in practice but remains a philosophical ideal. Its manifestations vary among cultures, among situations, and, most certainly, within one individual, depending on circumstances and with whom the relationship involving autonomy is created. Part of one's basic right to autonomy and self-determination is the right to refuse to exercise it and to ask for help and support in decision-making.

The legal system does not require absolute autonomy for any patient in this situation. In fact, the law concerning the relationship between physician and patient imposes a fiduciary relationship on the physician, who thus may not act toward the patient in any such arm's length way as would be demanded by the absolute autonomy of the patient.

In a fiduciary relationship one person is dealing with another under circumstances of special confidence; the person consulted has information or skills the other requires, and the beneficiary in the relationship by definition is unable to protect his or her own interests. The fiduciary is bound to act in good faith and with due regard to all the interests of the person who has bestowed the confidence.[1] Historically, the three great professions of law, medicine, and theology conferred by acceptance into their professions this obligation on their members; nowadays only the members of those three professions are automatically held to that legal standard, but other, less formal relationships may also demand such trust.

The concept of fiduciary relationships began in the law of trusts, and the principles establishing the trustee's duties to the beneficiary are still very much a part of the law. The concepts date from at least as early as 13th-century English law, and the first recorded donation under a trust occurred in 1225.[2] The same obligations of loyalty, good faith, and fair play are still part of a fiduciary obligation in 1987. As Justice Cardozo[3] wrote, "The great rule of law . . . which holds a trustee to the duty of constant and unqualified loyalty is not a thing of forms and phrases."

Throughout the centuries, part of a fiduciary's obligation has been a duty of full disclosure. This obligation did not suddenly become a part of the law of the physician-patient relationship in 1957 when a court first used the term "informed consent."[4] When a physician deals with a patient or with a research subject, he or she as a fiduciary is obligated to make affirmative disclosures even if the patient does not ask questions. By contrast, the person who sells goods may not lie to a customer in response to a direct question about the condition of the merchandise, but if the prospective buyer does not ask, there is no duty to disclose. Therefore, historically (and long before Kant and Mill) there was a difference between the relationship of a physician and a patient and that between a used brougham salesman and a prospective buyer.

Having made all relevant information known to the beneficiary of the relationship, the fiduciary's duty of loyalty then requires him or her to continue to act with "the utmost frankness and fair play." This is, of course, the antithesis of a relationship based solely on the autonomy of the beneficiary or patient who, by definition in a fiduciary situation, has insufficient knowledge to protect his or her own best interests. The fiduciary relationship thus entirely precludes arm's length relationships.

Similarly, the patient hopes for more than an arm's length relationship with his or her physician. Because I expect to receive information about medical alternatives does not mean that I expect to choose among those alternatives with my life at stake as if I were buying a skirt at the store. For one thing, in addition to any legal obligations my physician may have as a fiduciary, I expect my physician to *care* if I live or die (and if she or he doesn't, I will take my problem elsewhere), and thus I expect my physician to behave as a reasonable human being. Part of being a reasonable human being in a crisis is offering the best advice—professional, intellectual, emotional, and plain human—one has to offer.

Lawyers and philosophers who advocate increasing respect for patients' decision-making authority do not ask for the shop-clerk approach to medical care, nor do they want it for themselves.

What then is "patient autonomy" in the mid-1980s? I question that it is what Dr. Duffy's article alleges it to be. A patient has a right to know what medical alternatives are reasonably available for the treatment of whatever problem the patient has; one assumes that means that the patient has the right to know what the problem is. The provision of information (informing) is, however, only one aspect of the transaction. Decision-making about illness (consenting) is not conducted as a theoretical or intellectual exercise. I doubt any sick person, even a lawyer, ever took refuge from terror or sought inspiration for making a treatment decision by reading *Critique of Pure Reason* or *Utilitarianism*.

Human beings have more than reason and intellect; human beings are emotional and social beings. Most people do not live in isolation, nor do they wish to. People have families, concerned friends, nosy aunts, fellow workers, and interested cousins. Many human relationships are messy and cantankerous, but they are real and they are important. Even the most autonomy-minded philosopher or lawyer presumably does not interact with his or her children, spouse, or nosy aunt solely at the intellectual arm's length level that theoretical autonomy requires, and any attempt to do so in a classroom or law office would have rendered him or her such an ineffective teacher or advocate that some employment other than philosophy or law would already have become necessary.

So while the informational stage of "autonomous" informed consent may be the discussion of a "menu" of treatments as Dr. Duffy suggests, the consenting aspects are a concept far removed from the abstract concepts of either Mill or Kant.

References

1. *Neagle v McMullen*, 334 Ill 168, 165 NE 605 (1929).
2. Pollack F, Maitland FW: *History of English Law, ed 2*. New York, Cambridge University Press, vol 2, 1959, pp 237–239.
3. *Globe Woolen Co v Utica Gas and Electric Co*, 224 NYS 2d 483 (1918).
4. *Salgo v Leland Stanford Board of Trustees*, 317 P2d 170 (Cal 1957).

Rebuttal: Negative
Thomas P. Duffy, M.D.

Professor Holder uses the example of skirt buying to define the limits of autonomy in the DPR. She omits mention of the virtual disappearance of good service, the inflated cost of quality merchandise, and the shoddy workmanship of most products in her skirt-purchasing experience. The wealthy consumer can still buy quality goods and pleasant services, although couture styles are not the fabric of most peoples' wardrobes. The standard consumer may be distressed by the decline in the garment industry, but most would agree that these are pedestrian concerns and of little note. Skirts are disposable items, part of the whim of each changing fashion season. Even if the buyer does not beware, the consequences for the buyer and society are minimal and unimportant. Not so unimportant are the implications of a parallel decline in the quality of the practice of medicine—one that may occur as the physician's role shifts in society.

The focus on autonomy has altered the expectations and behavior of patients and doctors in the DPR; many patients and physicians now hold consumerist views. Medicine was never free of the marketplace, but the concerns of the latter now play a larger and larger role in the DPR. An adversarial style has become more pervasive, with less and less paternalism—an expected response to patients' assertiveness about their right to control their own care. Unfortunately, the prohibition against acting for the benefit of another person's welfare without their knowledge (paternalism) may give way to atrophy in acting to benefit another person with their knowledge (beneficence). The critical fulcrum of the DPR, beneficence, may weaken as the profession becomes more and more a trade.

Professor Holder might see this as a minor threat because the profession has a fiduciary relationship of trust with its patients. Maintaining such trust has become the problem now that doctors no longer know best and patients are skeptical of physicians' traditional claims. A consumerist view by the patient invites a seller's view by the physician. Trust in the DPR depends on the patient's participation as much as the doctor's. When the patient unilaterally decides to reject the doctor's prescription, this action has the same implication for the erosion of the DPR as the physician acting without informed consent. The depiction of the DPR as an adversarial relationship wherein the physician attacks the autonomy of the patient has created a climate of mistrust in the practice of medicine, a climate initially begotten by medicine itself with its callous disregard of patients' rights and subsequently sustained by lawyers' restricted focus on these rights as the most important component of the DPR.

The disarray that now exists in the DPR should serve as a gadfly to the profession to reexamine and reassert the proper role of the physician. Professor Holder is correct in suggesting that physicians need to relate to patients as teachers to their students; the derivation of the word doctor is from docēre, to teach. As a doctor, one attempts to lead the patient out of illness, with instructions regarding the pathways that led to the disease and the journey necessary to restore health. An adversarial slant to the partnership is obviously counterproductive. Trust is central in the undertaking, with successful outcome attainable only if knowledge and wisdom are joined with kindness and respect for the person in need. Autonomy as the ultimate value in the DPR has diverted attention from this generosity of spirit with which the physician must attend the sick. If this generosity sometimes takes the guise of paternalism, it is an acceptable trade-off only if no threat to mutual trust is created by the action.

The DPR has shifting emphases, dictated by the many variables in the sick state; an intensive care unit is very different from a well-baby clinic. In whatever setting, the patient and physician must attempt to weigh the benefits and burdens of any decision. Legal and ethical guidelines will be exactly that—they will help to guide the profession in recognizing and dissecting the problem. The solutions must come from the medical profession, acting in good conscience to ensure the proper outcome of medical care. This will encompass respect for autonomy and informed consent together with the challenge to recognize the unique needs of each patient.

Editor's Comments
Gary Gitnick, M.D.

Rarely in the day-to-day practice of modern medicine do we take time to ponder the social and attitudinal changes that are reflected in our current approaches to patient care. The debate before us questions whether patient autonomy eliminates any role for paternalism in a DPR.

To this question, Ms. Holder firmly states that a role for paternalism no longer exists. She carefully traces the gradual alterations that have occurred in the relative roles of men and women, husbands and wives, children and parents, patients and doctors over the past 15 years. The historical development of our modern concept of informed consent eventually altered significantly the attitudes of physicians and patients and established the concept of patient autonomy. She emphatically defends her contention that paternalism no longer has a role in modern American medical practice.

She emphasizes that the last 15 years have brought the American public to believe patients are entitled to be taught to understand and to make decisions that previously were made for them by their physicians. In her view, the role of the physician is to provide advice and help but not to violate the autonomy of the patient to make the final decision after being properly informed.

In contrast, Dr. Duffy upholds the concept of paternalism in medicine while still defending the patient's right to be informed and at least to join in the decision-making process. He argues that the patient deprives himself of a significant ally when he denies the decision-making process to the physician. He points out that patients, no matter how well informed by physicians and other advisers, can easily make fatal decisions because of inadequate background and experience. An unjustified fear of discomfort or inability to see beyond the immediate problem may obscure the long-term promise of cure and comfort. The patient's ability to decide may be altered by illness and may lead to a distorted assessment of the illness, especially for someone who is experiencing a life-threatening illness or who has never been involved in illness among friends, relatives, or self (the most common situation for society at present). In declining appropriate treatment, patients may actually cause themselves harm. He points out that illness may take a toll of emotional reserves, may preclude clear and considered thinking, and may result in distorted views and improper determinations.

He further points out that the physician who serves as friend and adviser to such a patient may be unable to educate the patient adequately in the choices that exist. This may lead to decisions to reject potentially helpful therapy. He points out that relegating the physician solely to the role of teacher or conveyer of information may lead to a generation of physicians who consider themselves purely as educators. No longer will patients benefit from the astute clinician who acts on the basis of clinical intuition and judgment developed through lengthy experience. Gone will be the physician who was willing to fight crisis after crisis in the hopes of a future cure. No longer will we consider the doctor in the role of "attending physician." The new role of the physician would be that of counselor. To these arguments Ms. Holder responds that everyone has the basic right to absolute autonomy and self-determination. They also have the right to relinquish self-determination and autonomy and to seek the support and decision-making abilities of a physician. It is up to the patient to decide whether to remain autonomous or to relegate decision-making to the physician.

Dr. Duffy asserts that the institution of the concept of patient autonomy often places the physician and patient in an adversarial role, a situation that may alter the traditional, beneficent physician-patient relationship. He agrees that physicians should serve as teachers to their patients, but he maintains that an adversarial relationship between teacher and student is counterproductive. The physician-patient relationship, he contends, must be based on trust and respect on the part of the patient, and wisdom, knowledge, kindness, and respect on the part of the physician.

Both discussants make valuable points and have justification. Modern medical practice has changed and will continue to evolve. The hospital need not become a courtroom. The challenges to the good physician are increasing. He or she may retire to the safety of the concept that physicians serve only to advise. He or she may master the greater art of medicine, which in the future will encompass roles not only as counselor, teacher, and guide but also as a person of great experience, knowledge, intuition, and expertise. These are qualities that patients should utilize. With luck, the art of medicine will blend with demands for patient autonomy to the greater benefit of physicians and patients.

Index

TO ORDER: DETACH AND MAIL

Please enter my subscription to the journal(s) and/or Year Book(s) checked below:
(To order by phone, call **toll-free 800-622-5410**. In IL, call **collect 312-726-9746**.)

	Practitioner (approx.)	Resident	Institution
Current Problems in Surgery® (1 yr.)	____$55.00	____$29.95	____$72.00
Current Problems in Pediatrics® (1 yr.)	____$39.95	____$29.95	____$65.00
Current Problems in Cancer® (1 yr.)	____$49.95	____$29.95	____$65.00
Current Problems in Cardiology® (1 yr.)	____$49.95	____$29.95	____$65.00
Current Problems in Obstetrics, Gynecology, and Fertility® (1 yr.)	____$49.95	____$29.95	____$65.00
Current Problems in Diag. Radiology® (1 yr.)	____$49.95	____$29.95	____$72.00
Disease-A-Month® (1 yr.)	____$39.95	____$29.95	____$65.00
	Binder____$14.95 (two-year)		
1988 Year Book of Anesthesia® (AN-88)	____$44.95	____$29.95	
1988 Year Book of Cancer® (CA-88)	____$44.95	____$29.95	
1988 Year Book of Cardiology® (CV-88)	____$44.95	____$29.95	
1988 Year Book of Critical Care Medicine®(16-88)	____$45.95	____$29.95	
1988 Year Book of Dentistry® (D-88)	____$45.95	____$29.95	
1988 Year Book of Dermatology® (10-88)	____$45.95	____$29.95	
1988 Year Book of Diagnostic Radiology® (9-88)	____$44.95	____$29.95	
1988 Year Book of Digestive Diseases (13-88)	____$42.95	____$29.95	
1988 Year Book of Drug Therapy (6-88)	____$44.95	____$29.95	
1988 Year Book of Emergency Medicine® (15-88)	____$44.95	____$29.95	
1988 Year Book of Endocrinology® (EM-88)	____$45.95	____$29.95	
1988 Year Book of Family Practice® (FY-88)	____$42.95	____$29.95	
1988 Year Book of Geriatrics and Gerontology (GE-88)	____$39.95	____$29.95	
1988 Year Book of Hand Surgery® (17-88)	____$42.95	____$29.95	
1988 Year Book of Hematology (24-88)	____$39.95	____$29.95	
1988 Year Book of Infectious Diseases (19-88)	____$39.95	____$29.95	
1988 Year Book of Medicine® (1-88)	____$44.95	____$29.95	
1988 Year Book of Neonatal/Perinatal Medicine (23-88)	____$42.95	____$29.95	
1988 Year Book of Neurology and Neurosurgery® (8-88)	____$44.95	____$29.95	
1988 Year Book of Nuclear Medicine® (NM-88)	____$45.00	____$29.95	
1988 Year Book of Obstetrics and Gynecology® (5-88)	____$42.95	____$29.95	
1988 Year Book of Ophthalmology® (EY-88)	____$44.95	____$29.95	
1988 Year Book of Orthopedics® (OR-88)	____$44.95	____$29.95	
1988 Year Book of Otolaryngology-Head and Neck Surgery (3-88)	____$44.95	____$29.95	
1988 Year Book of Pathology and Clinical Pathology® (PI-88)	____$44.95	____$29.95	
1988 Year Book of Pediatrics® (4-88)	____$42.95	____$29.95	
1988 Year Book of Plastic and Reconstructive Surgery® (12-88)	____$46.95	____$29.95	
1988 Year Book of Podiatric Medicine and Surgery (18-88)	____$42.95	____$29.95	
1988 Year Book of Psychiatry and Applied Mental Health® (11-88)	____$42.95	____$29.95	
1988 Year Book of Pulmonary Disease (21-88)	____$42.95	____$29.95	
1988 Year Book of Rehabilitation (22-88)	____$42.95	____$29.95	
1988 Year Book of Sports Medicine® (SM-88)	____$42.95	____$29.95	
1988 Year Book of Surgery® (2-88)	____$47.95	____$29.95	
1988 Year Book of Urology® (7-88)	____$44.95	____$29.95	
1988 Year Book of Vascular Surgery (20-88)	____$42.95	____$29.95	

NAME_____ACCT. NO._____

ADDRESS_____

CITY_____STATE_____ZIP_____

Printed in U.S.A.   DFI

YEAR BOOK MEDICAL PUBLISHERS
35 EAST WACKER DRIVE   CHICAGO, ILLINOIS 60601